Medical Tourism

Surgery for Sale!

How to Have Surgery Abroad Without It Costing Your Life

JANET BRISTEIR

ISBN - 13: 978-0-9970968-0-4
ISBN - 10: 0-9970968-0-2

This publication is designed to provide accurate and authoritative information in regard to the subject matter covered. It is sold with the understanding that the publisher is not engaged in rendering medical, legal, accounting, or other professional services.

If medical advice or other expert assistance is required, the services of a competent professional person should be sought.

Published by: Celebrity Expert Author
http://celebrityexpertauthor.com

Canadian Address:	US Address:
Celebrity Expert Author	1300 Boblett Street
501- 1155 The High Street,	Unit A-218
Coquitlam, BC, Canada	Blaine, WA 98230
V3B.7W4	Phone: (866) 492-6623
Phone: (604) 941-3041	Fax: (250) 493-6603
Fax: (604) 944-7993	

Table of Contents

Checklists available at: areusafe.ca
Medical Tourism Facilitator (MTF) Checklist
Checklist of Cost Factors to Consider
Checklist for Facility
Questions to Ask the Surgeon
26 Pre surgery Checklist questions

Introduction

IN AUGUST 2015 the first Canadian Medical Tourism tradeshow was held in Montreal, Quebec. In the tradeshow information package they had the following statistics:

1) Over 800,000 Canadians travel outside the country on a yearly basis to obtain medical/dental services not pre-approved by their provincial health plan.

2) In 2014, Canadian Medical Tourism increased by 26%.

3) Canadians are spending over $400,000,000 USD per year since 2009 for out-of-country medical services.

Introduction to Medical Tourism

When people speak of medical tourism they are usually discussing the practice of going outside of the country where they live and paying for a surgical procedure to be performed.

The surgery can be a procedure they either need or want however, for some reason they are prevented from having the surgery at home. There are numerous reasons that the surgery may not be available:

- The surgery is not performed in the country.
- They are not perceived by their doctor as a candidate for this procedure.

- There may be a long waiting list for the surgery which they don't want to endure.

Overall, people arrive at a decision to investigate Medical Tourism for a number of reasons. Medical tourism can be a great decision and provide the desired outcome.

The purpose of this book is to help you see the big picture of the decision you are making if you are considering having surgery abroad and to allow you to weigh as many factors as possible to help you achieve the best possible outcome. You can get your desired outcome if you keep your expectations within an achievable range. I am reminded of the old joke: *A patient was having hand surgery and asked the doctor if he would be able to play the piano. The doctor said, yes, the patient said, great I couldn't play before!*

Medical tourism is easily found in mainstream media these days; a Google search will give you 27,200,000 hits for the topic.

In the film, "The Best Exotic Marigold Hotel", Maggie Smith plays an elderly woman who travels from the UK to India for hip surgery. She's sent by the National Health Service, as part of their program to reduce wait times for surgery.

There's an "Idiots Guide to Medical Tourism" book.

There's a book written by a man who helped his cousin seek a kidney transplant in China, "Larry's Kidney" by Daniel Asa Rose.

All the information is diverse and can be overwhelming.

What is Medical Tourism?

The Fraser Institute published a report in March 2015 which stated:

"In 2014, an estimated 52,513 Canadians received non-emergency medical treatment outside Canada. In some cases, these patients needed to leave Canada due to a lack of available resources or a lack of appropriate procedures or technologies. In others, their departure will have been driven by a desire to return more quickly to their lives, to seek out superior quality care, or perhaps to save their own lives or avoid the risk of disability."

At the time of needing to have surgery or making the decision to have surgery most people's expectations of the medical system are based on what they see on TV. When you are the person initiating the decision to have the surgery in another country, you are not just being plugged into a healthcare system; you are also traveling to another country, possibly another culture. You are the sole person making many decisions that affect your outcome.

In Canada we take things for granted within the healthcare system and we believe what people tell us about the process and expected outcome of our surgery. Before you commit to any procedure, you should be aware of the fact that there are a lot of things that go on in the background that the average person doesn't think about related to a surgical procedure whether it a minor or major procedure.

Your belief in the decision and its positive outcome when you embark on this proactive endeavor makes a positive outcome possible.

What is the best possible outcome?

- Feeling good about yourself

- Positive body image; the way that you see yourself
- Function; expectations of what you can and can't do
  - o Alignment between expectation and outcome; when it's not there, you set yourself up for failure
- You feel good about your decision
- You have support from your family and friends
- You know how to proceed so that feel good about yourself
- You are in control, empowered to live to your full capacity

If you have support, belief, alignment and expectation around the outcome, you will get a better result from your surgery. If you are considering Medical Tourism there are critical elements needed to provide you with a successful medical tourism experience.

You can get a good outcome with medical tourism when you understand the **5 Critical Elements** related to the best possible outcome.

1) Motivating factors for wanting surgery; are there limitations in our healthcare system
   a) Is it a necessity
   b) Is your desire
   c) What are your reasons for looking abroad
   d) What are the unseen factors
   e) Have you considered all the options
   f) Have you thought through why you want what you want
   g) Do you have support and agreement from family and friends

      h) Do you have support and agreement of your doctor

      i) Have you evaluated the reality of the decision

2) Evaluation of the best and safest options (Action plan)

      a) How are you choosing where you want to go

      b) Do you have relatives and family ties in the area

      c) Is it based on a destination you have always wanted to visit

      d) What research have you done

      e) Do you know what costs are involved; the real and total cost

      f) Have you considered letting someone who knows the process book it for you

      g) Are you comfortable making travel arrangements and speaking to health care professionals

3) **Getting it done, following through on the plan, making the experience as smooth as possible.**
These are some of the things to consider when making your plans:

Factoring in pre-surgery requirements, travel time and recovery time

      a) Time off work for you and your companion

      b) Travel

      c) Insurance

  d) Timing

  e) After care

  f) Medications

  g) Recovery time

  h) Support and companionship

  i) Vacation

  j) Logistics

4) Coming home; ensuring the best possible outcome

  a) Medical support in this country

  b) Follow up

  c) Medication

  d) Reintegration into our healthcare

  e) Recovery

  f) Rehab

  g) Additional surgeries

  h) Insurance coverage

  i) Recovery time off work

  j) What if there's a complication

In this book we will explore the 5 Critical Elements you need to consider when contemplating paying for surgery abroad.

Element One: The Motivating Factors for Wanting Surgery

PEOPLE LOOKING FOR surgery abroad are as varied as the conditions and reasons they are researching for surgery. When you consider surgery abroad there can be a number of influencing factors: mobility, activity, lifestyle, whether the condition is life-threatening, your self-esteem, and your self-confidence. Is your quality of life reduced due to constant pain and immobility?

Factors that are affecting lifestyle or mobility

There are various groups of people looking at paying for surgery abroad; the groups could depend on a particular condition or required surgery. There are people looking for orthopaedic surgeries; people who have Multiple Sclerosis who are looking at a **liberation procedure**; people with weight challenges investigating bariatric surgery (a gastric procedure that reduces the size of the stomach) or it might be dental or cosmetic surgery. It might be the inability to eat properly because they need a dental procedure. They could be having difficulty losing weight causing lack of mobility which in itself can be increasing the incidence of other health problems such as heart disease, Diabetes Mellitus, many types of cancer, Asthma, sleep apnea, and chronic musculo-skeletal problems there are several health factors that come into decreased mobility and have an influences on lifestyle.

Liberation procedure is the term used for an endovascular surgery. It involves placing a tiny balloon or tube called a stent inside a blocked vein to open it and restore blood flow out of the brain and spinal cord. The procedure is used for the treatment for CCSVI which stands for Chronic Cerebrospinal Venous Insufficiency, which is a narrowing of veins in the neck and chest that carry blood away from the brain and spinal cord. Researchers have been studying whether treating CCSVI by opening up blocked veins can improve symptoms caused by MS.

Conditions that are life-threatening, or that might threaten longevity.

The discussion around solid organ transplants abroad brings many legal and ethical questions to the surface. It is not so main-stream because when you start discussing whether someone is going to get an organ in another country there are restrictions and ethical considerations. Where is the organ coming from? How was the donor screened for a match to the recipient? What follow-up care does the donor receive? How much does the donor receive? These would be a few of the biggest questions.

It's a very different scenario if you are 72 years old and you are given a two year wait for your knee replacement. You might have a really active lifestyle however, because of your age you are put at the bottom of the list. You want to maintain your active lifestyle, to be able to play with the great-grand-children, play a round of golf or just be self-sufficient. Why should you be restricted for two years if you have the money and the time to go and have surgery abroad that obviously will enhance your life?

Self-esteem and confidence: what kind of surgeries are people looking for abroad?

The main surgery in the media at present regarding confidence and self-esteem is probably bariatric surgery. There's a lot of media attention on obesity, every magazine at the supermarket has the latest diet fad or details of a well know personalities loss or gain on a diet. Obesity and overweight are used interchangeably; a common definition being of a Body Mass Index (BMI) of between 25 -30. (BMI is calculated by taking the persons weight and dividing by the square of their height.)

When we talk of bariatric surgery patients it could be someone's who is 350 - 400 pounds or more. They have tried every diet under the sun and their weight fluctuates back and forth. They may have seen articles about these surgeries that will reduce their stomach capacity and will help them with their weight-loss. People are looking to regain self-esteem and confidence with weight-loss that they've not been able to manage on their own up to this point.

There are also plastic surgeries, liposuction where people have fat removed from the abdomen, thighs and buttocks. Once we enter into plastic or cosmetic surgery there are a multitude of reasons people feel that they need surgeries for cosmetic reasons. Looking at them, you might think, "I don't know why they need that," however to them, it's something that's playing on their mind every day all day. It has a big effect on their life.

The increase in teenagers asking for plastic surgery may see a trend of teens having surgery combined with their vacations:

In the USA according to American Society of Plastic Surgeons (ASPS) statistics, 63,623 cosmetic surgical procedures were performed on people age 13-19 in 2013, while 155,941 cosmetic minimally-invasive procedures were performed.

The New York Post stated that 18,000 American teens got Botox in one form or another in 2013.

An article in the Vancouver 24hrs newspaper in August 2015 stated that "The Teen plastic surgery boom is being driven by our obsession with all things celebrity".

In the UK the National Health Service reported in 2013 that when interviewed 60 % of girls aged 11 – 16 said they felt some pressure to look the way celebrities do.

Magazines and advertising play into feelings of low esteem, to how someone feels about themselves and this will affect their decision about whether to have surgery or why they can't have it. If someone feels that they have a physical deficit, and all the TV, all the magazines, all media plays into "this is the perfect image," it's reinforcing that, over and over again. If you have the time and the money to choose to go for cosmetic surgery abroad it is going to be a seriously considered option. Depending on the surgery there will still need to be work on the psychological aspect of the change, just because you have the surgery doesn't mean that the mental image that you have of yourself is going to change.

Quality of Life and Pain.
What motivates people?

Quality of life and pain are huge motivators. Bariatric surgery can be prescribed in the Canadian Health care system however, I've heard of people waiting up to 6- 8 years for the surgery. While they were waiting maybe other medical conditions could creep into their lives; such as heart disease, diabetes mellitus, cancer, asthma, sleep apnea, and chronic musculoskeletal problems.

If you are waiting for two years to get hip or knee surgery your mobility and reliability on painkillers affects you every moment of your day. You are not as mobile as you might be there is the possibility that your health is going to deteriorate over the years you are waiting. If you have something wrong with your joints, you are not walking so well. If it's your shoulder, you can't lift things, you can't dress yourself properly. It's all of these day-to-day activities, needing pain management , which can affect your ability to do other things. Depending on what you are not able to do, it affects your mental state as well. If you are in pain, you are not the bright and cheery person that you could be.

Patient Motivation: It's time to do
something about this!

People get to a point where they are motivated. Where it is just time to do something about the condition that is affecting them. You may see an article in a magazine or see a new procedure on the TV. Something changes, you either come to a point of "I can't stand this anymore; I'm going to do something about it myself," or "Oh, look! It's available here. I could probably get there and do that." Something shifts, and that moves you forward with your decision of, "Yes, I'm going to look into this." I want to make a change in my life now.

An example I can give you related to dental treatments:

MK had problems with her gums and was told by a dentist that she needed 3 or 4 teeth extracted and should be having 3 monthly examinations and cleaning due to bad gingivitis (inflammation of the gums around the roots of the teeth). Although MK knew this was an excellent dentist, (it was actually the second time she'd been told she needed to have treatment regarding her gums and loose teeth) the treatment was going to cost about $9,000 and she couldn't bring herself to commit to the suggested course of treatment. MK and her husband are Canadian Snow Birds; they spend the winter months in Mexico. From her conversations with other Snow Birds and American friends MK knew there were dentists in Mexico that were very economical. Five years after MKs visit to the Canadian dentists she decided the time had come and she was going to have the procedures done in the Baja, California, in a town called Los Algodones, which has about 90 dental offices catering to cross border patients.

As MK did not have a referral from a dentist or friend at this time, she took to the internet to research dentists on her own. Having decided on the dentist she liked MK arranged to go and have the treatments in Los Algodones. She was very pleased with the outcome, she didn't have any teeth removed, but had extensive work; 3 laser cleanings, 4 root canals, and extensive crown work in a three week period. It had taken her five years to get to the decision to have the treatments abroad and once there she committed to a much more extensive dental treatment plan in a relatively short period of time (three weeks).

The Wait Time, the Mobility, and Activity Level, Possible Deterioration.

These factors will affect the level of urgency you feel. It might be you have got the children's graduation coming up, a wedding, a high school reunion; an important occasion that's ahead and if you don't get something done about your condition; you won't be able to participate in it. There are all kinds of things that motivate people. Basically the medical system isn't fitting into the timeframe of your life. It's stopping you moving on with your life.

Timing: the Window of Opportunity for Getting Surgery.

It might be that with the physical restrictions of your condition's you are off work. However, you won't be covered by the health plan for the extended wait period, so this surgery needs to be done now. It might be that you have had some kind of change in circumstance that you now have a window of opportunity. Perhaps you are between jobs, or a contract has finished, something that gives you the chance to go and get the surgery done. Perhaps the person who's going to be your caregiver is available at this point in time and they haven't been available before. A window of opportunity can present itself and move the decision for surgery abroad forward when least expected.

You may have considered blending the surgery with wanting to visit a particular country, to have a vacation after the surgery. Or it might be that if you are from another country, you choose to go back to your country of origin since you know the surgery will cost less there. You may be able to take an extended holiday, where you'll have the surgery, and you'll have family there to look after you.

Feeling Like Time Is Running Out.

This is probably a big factor, there are so many times you can consider this, it could be younger people with mobility issues wanting to be active or older people at different peak stages in their lives.

It might not be someone in their 50's, 60's, looking for a round of golf. Actually some people in their mid-20s might have problems with their joints that require surgery. If you are in your 20's you might be thinking "I don't want to wait for this surgery; I want to get this fixed, I missing out on X, Y, Z, that all my friends are doing, or an opportunity to travel or to work abroad." These are contributing factors; as well as the pressure to search for "instant gratification" that we all are subjected to constantly by the media. So the dilemma becomes why would you, why should you wait for this surgery?

You might look at it like having something repaired on the car. The thought that getting a part replaced, just getting that replacement part put in your knee, is going to make all the difference, and you'll be able to walk again. Those factors are really important as people age, too, because we all know that phrase "you use it or lose it" the longer you are out of practice doing something, the harder it will be to get back to the life desired.

We also have a longer lifespan. In my parents' time, when they were in their 60's, if they went to their G.P. and said something was hurting, they would be told, "Well, what do you expect at your age?" Now I'm 60; if someone told me, "What do you expect at your age?" I would tell them exactly what I expected! Our expectations are much different than our parents. Maybe at 80 or 85 someone could say, "What do you expect at your age?" however not to a person in their early 60's. Healthcare practicioners are finding that there are a lot of people who are not prepared to settle into the armchair and let life go by anymore.

Emotional Motivations: Fear, Time, Money, and Suffering.

Fear and Pain

Pain is something that plays such a big part in some people's life. If you wake up in the morning and you are in pain, that sets the pace for your day; what if you can't get out of bed because you are in pain? There's that fear when you first wake up, "What if I can't move? What if this doesn't stop?" The pain controls how can function while carrying out your daily living activities. It might also be that there is a medication you are taking that's controlling the pain, but reducing your abilities to do other things. There might be side effects from the painkillers: gastric side effects, difficulty eating, and problems with change in bowel activity. There may be sedation side effects where you become drowsy or shouldn't be driving or operating machinery. With constant pain you could be watching your life shrink around you. It can limit your mobility and can make you depressed. There's the chance that you will irritable most of the time because of your pain, so your friends are going to stop phoning. It's not easy for them to phone, to say, "I'm going to drop by," or "Let me take you out for lunch." because when they do you are grumbling and moaning about the pain and there's nothing they can do about itand this makes them feel inadequate. Your circle of friends is likely to get smaller and you are going to be more isolated, giving you more time to dwell on your pain.

Pain can affect your ability to participate: in the family, social or physical activities; if you do manage to get to a family event or a social activity and you are in pain, you are wary that someone's going to come by and knock your knee or hurt your elbow whatever is the focus of your pain, so you are on high alert all the time. And that, again, doesn't add to your social skills.

I mentioned bariatric surgery earlier. A lot of the clientele for stomach reduction surgeries are women and men that have younger children, they are thinking, "I want to be able to participate fully in my child's life. Unless I do something now, I'm not going to be able to do that." This can be a different sort of social isolation as the children get older and do not want an obese parent to attend school functions for fear of what their peers may say and tease them about at school.

Self-Esteem and Feeling Less Than

Self-esteem and feeling "less than" can be particularly highlighted if you are a parent. All children go through a stage where they don't want to be seen with their parents however children with parents who are overweight will often say, "Don't drop me off outside the school," or "Don't come to this," or "Don't come to that." They feel that the other kids are going to laugh at them. Self-esteem is a big motivating factor in the medical tourism industry. Wanting to take part in the children's activities can be the deciding factor in someone's decision to investigate bariatric surgery options.

Being overweight a can bring along mobility issues. The lack of mobility can compound other medical conditions which can affect your heart, respiratory, gastric systems and also can create problems with joints. If you can't get around, you have to depend on other people helping you. Your family and friends have to do more as you can't participate in general daily living activities as much as you'd like to. You have to rely on the family doing more of the chores; cleaning, laundry, getting shopping, and cooking for you. Your self-esteem is reduced and you get that feeling of being less than you used to be.

In Canada, because our healthcare is socialized, we do have access to a variety of bariatric and cosmetic surgeries however, they rank low in the necessity scale. You can get bariatric surgery in the Canadian healthcare system; if you get above a certain weight, if you fit into the criteria, if you jump through all the hoops that are deemed necessary. I have been told the process can take six to eight years depending where you live Canada. That six or eight years is part of the child's life that you are not able to participate in fully. If someone offered you the chance to have the surgery today, you'd probably do all you could to go and have it.

Sense of Loss and Loss of Ability

People can feel a sense of loss. It's that feeling that they are missing out of doing things, going places, participating.

As I said before, loss of ability, "use it or lose it." If you are not walking, or if you have something wrong with your shoulder, if you are not using your arms properly, it will all take time to build it up again. You might not even be aware of the loss until you are going to do something that's commonplace: open a door or stand up or kneel down to pick something up off the floor, it's that, "Oh, I can't do that now." And finally you think what do I do now?

The advent of Medical Tourism opens the door to the idea of you being able to have more control over surgeries of what's being done to your body. You might almost feel you have a chance, more say, or more ability to do something to recover a function that you thought was long gone, lost forever.

We have different expectations these days when it comes to what we will or won't endure, even without medical tourism. I was talking to someone recently who was very pregnant. She's quite petite, she still had a month to go and the baby is seven plus pounds, and she told me, "I booked a Caesarean section. I'm not going through a natural birth with a potentially eight pound plus baby!" We have the choice these days, and the regular mind-set that we can choose what happens to our bodies.

Hopelessness and Loss of Control

If you have been told you have three years to wait for surgery, and there's nothing else in the meantime apart from painkillers, loss of mobility and the isolation. Or if you have been told, "Yes, you may be a candidate for bariatric surgery, however you have to do this, see this consultant, go on this diet, and we'll let you know if you'll be considered". It's that not having control of the action plan. If you opt for surgery abroad, you are being pro-active, not passive. You are taking things into your hands building up your self-esteem and moving forward to a resolution of the problem. There's still a timeframe of things you need to do, however once things start rolling you will feel there is movement forward, action happening, and it can cause a big shift in your outlook, to your energy and things can start to look more hopeful.

It's similar to having something to look forward to in the winter; people have holidays in January or February just to get themselves through those dark months. If you were sitting waiting for a surgery for two years, and then you made a decision to have the surgery abroad, you could be thinking, "Oh, this is going to happen next month," it really changes your whole perspective and that can have a big impact on your wellbeing.

How Has Your Life Changed Because Of This Problem?

We all have a sense of who we are, which might not be the perception that other people have of us however, if someone has been very active and suddenly something's wrong with their joints, they are not able to play golf or garden, so they cut that out of their routine. They can't go for the walks that they used to have, they are sitting around more, this causes them to stiffen up more, use it or lose it again. This plays on their sense of who they are. It could be someone who is constantly on different diets, trying to lose weight, it's just not happening, and they are doing everything that they feel that they can. It's these scenarios play into the sense of who you are. Maybe you are considering a cosmetic surgery; you see a part of you that you find flawed, you see it in the mirror every day, probably no-one else notices it however, to you, that's who you are, and if it was fixed, it would make a huge difference to your sense of self. Your life would be different if only this surgery could take place a quickly as possible.

Support of Family and Friends

Having a supportive family and group of friends can be a huge contributing factor in your mental and physical well-being. Is your family supportive? With this loss of ability, loss of mobility, is your family supporting you? Are you getting that help that you need at home? Do they understand tt you have limitations now? If you are going on diets trying to lose weight, do they understand you are trying to keep on this diet and not just saying, "Oh, just have one of these it won't hurt?" What support do you actually get at home? And how does that affect the home life and how you carry on with the regime you have set yourself?

Contribution and participation to home life could also be a big factor. If you have a problem with your joints or you are overweight, can you participate in the household chores? Who is covering the chores that you can no longer perform? Does that build up resentment? How is this lack of mobility affecting your relationship with your partner, or your children? If you are off work, are you losing money because you are off work? How does that play into the family dynamic?

Fear of Losing Income

Depending on the physical problem you have, there may come a time when you can't work. When you are not able to physically do the job, or the painkillers you take reduce your ability to operate the machinery or concentrate on your work. You might have a very physically demanding job and the company can't accommodate you with a less physical job, so you might be on extended leave while you are waiting for surgery. Hopefully you have health benefits that would kick in, however if you don't, where does the money come from? This will add stress to you and your immediate family and the dynamics within it; which might be the catalyst that prompts you to go overbroad for surgery so you can continue to work.

Quality of Life and Leisure Activities.

We all have high expectations which are fed to us by the media, whether it's TV, print, film; that people should be engaged in some kind of leisure activities. We know that this could be as simple as the grandkids coming to visit and you can play with them or take them to the park. There can be a sport you participate in, a walking group, a reading group. These all take time, money and mobility to participate in. If you are having problems with pain and mobility, or you have a reduced income because of being unable to work you will not be able to pursue these. Perhaps the next time you see in the media the availability of surgeries abroad, you will be more receptive to the idea and it will now play a role in making a decision about the possibility of you, having your surgery abroad.

The media also publicises increased activity levels and more extreme sports which introduces a lot of younger people to the need for surgeries. There could also be a younger group of surgery seekers with conditions like MS that are going for liberation surgery. The age range for people seeking surgery abroad has been quoted as between 22 and 80 years of age.

Desire: Life with the Perfect Outcome.

With a lot of surgeries, people are looking for a quick fix, the instant gratification I spoke of earlier. There is an expectation that the surgery is going to be a magic wand, everything will be OK once the surgery have been completed.

It is what we are exposed to all the time on the TV shows. The reality is that whatever surgery you have there is work involved for you. It may appear that when you are looking at orthopaedic surgery, your knee or your hip for instance, that's very mechanical, a bit like getting a car fixed. This joint's not working; we're going to replace it. The new joint will work however, you'll still have to do the work, make sure that you are building up the muscles and flexibility and helping with the healing that occurs afterward. It's not going to be instant; however, it definitely has the potential to change your life for the better.

It's the same with bariatric surgery. Yes, the surgery will reduce the capacity of the food your stomach can deal with however, there's still going to a lot be work that you'll have to do afterwards. You are not going to go in to that surgery at 400 pounds and come out at 200. There is still engagement and commitment in the process you have to make to get the perfect outcome you are expecting, however, definitely the potential is there. You will have to be committed to a new lifestyle, to changes in eating habits, regular exercise routines, to have a new perspective on what you can accomplish.

People are More Engaged in Life.

I heard this acronym used a while ago which sums up what is important in people's lives; **F.O.R.M.**: Family, Occupation, Recreation, and Motivation. We all want to be fully engaged, we are motivated to be involved with our family, our occupation and our recreational activities. If you have a debilitating condition which in effect removes you from being engaged in these activities your world becomes narrower, you are limited in what you can do. Surgery holds out the "carrot". You are hoping to be living a different life when they get back from surgery, fully engaged again and motivated to move forward with your life.

The decision to travel abroad and have surgery will be life changing. There will be the physical relief that the surgery will bring you, also the sense of achievement that you have taken control, travelled to another country, got your life back on track. The fact of travelling abroad will change your impression of the world; hopefully for the better. You will experience a different country, maybe a different culture during and after surgery. You will possibly have time to visit tourist attractions near the health facility where you have your surgery. Ultimately, taking action and making something happen continues to have positive a effect on your healing after the surgery.

Psychologically, if you go into something, you are taking control of it, you are visualizing "This is going to make me better; I'm going to be mobile; It is going to help me lose weight," you have got a psychological edge that really helps your healing. It's a very positive attitude to be in control, to be planning to move forward. "This is the outcome I'm expecting, this is going to happen." It will help with achieving the desired end result and help create a more optimistic environment for you, your family, everyone in your immediate social circle.

Happier, fulfilled, and achieving your potential.

The decision to have surgery abroad could bring about a major shift in your life.

One of the people interviewed about bariatric surgery,

had a major change in her life after the surgery. She went to have bariatric surgery in Mexico, and was so pleased with the outcome that she asked the surgeon if she could work with him and help other people who needed bariatric surgery by referring them to him. She has taken courses in counselling and nutrition, she's also trained as a Medical Tourism Facilitator. She gave up her job and now is a full time medical tourism facilitator for that facility. Her service for bariatric patients provides pre and post-surgery counselling and support groups. Her decision to have surgery abroad completely changed her life. Not only did she achieve the outcome she envisioned, she has also unleashed her potential to help others achieve their goals.

Ability, Mobility, Activity, and Self-Sufficiency.

If you have had loss of mobility that has affected your ability to participate fully in life, you are much more motivated to get that mobility back. You will push yourself further than you did before as you now don't take things for granted. Once you have lost something, if you have an opportunity to get it back again, you really use it. I believe that people who are motivated to get their surgeries aboard have the potential to be much more active in their recovery phase. You will go to the physiotherapist, do the exercises, and you are going to follow the eating plan. You will be really engaged in it and not reliant on someone else telling you what to do next; waiting for the silver bullet to fix it. Your attitude is going to be more positive; "Okay, this is what I can do today; what do I have to do to be able to do this and more tomorrow?"

Many surgeries require physiotherapy post operatively. It may be prescribed to go to physiotherapist three times a week, as part of their rehabilitation program. People at home relying on the healthcare system can make all kinds of excuses not to go to appointments or do the exercises. They are not feeling so good, "Oh, perhaps I'll do it another day." I can catch up when I feel better. However if you get into this process yourself; you have gone abroad, had surgery, and you know that physiotherapy three times a week, plus following the exercise plan is going to get you to where you want to be physically, you are going to do it. You will be more engaged to achieve self-sufficiency.

Comfort, Relief, Emotional Wellbeing, and Decreased Stress

The overall effect on someone's wellbeing works on so many levels The image you have been carrying with you of what you will be able to do if you lost weight or if you looked different, if you have that physical change, is now a reality. There will be the relief that it's actually been done and you can move on to the next part of your life. Emotionally, you will feel that release and that will help you engage more with family, friends, and return to work. This will definitely decrease the stress. Also if you are not in pain, you are not going to be as stressed as you were before.

Medical tourism is a topic that has come more and more into the public's awareness, especially with the change in healthcare in the United States. In the States the insurance companies are now embracing medical tourism because they can often get a better deal abroad than they can in country.

It's also affecting travel patterns of Americans. I read that 40 % of the people in the States don't have a passport, and haven't travelled outside their home State. Suddenly you have a group of people who might need surgery who are being told, "If you go abroad and have this surgery under this insurance plan, you can have your surgery next week, and we'll give you a thousand dollars for going, and you'll be back at work faster than expected." It's a very interesting phenomenon; people who have never considered traveling outside of their State are now going to be exposed to different cultures and experiences due to medical tourism.

More and more stories of medical tourism are coming into the media as well, which raises the profile of medical tourism for people elsewhere, and makes them consider that this might be a possibility for the surgery they need. If insurance companies in America are thinking about sending clients abroad for surgery, it must be a good deal, mustn't it? People who have been on waiting lists or wanting surgery will perhaps now be thinking; "I'll look into this, I might be able to do it, save some money and get my surgery faster".

Insurance companies are always looking for the most economical way to fulfil their policy claims. I think that will also happen with Canadian health insurance companies. If people have private health insurance, companies will definitely be looking for any significant saving they can make by sending clients out of the country.

The other thing that is happening in the States and on the medical tourism websites is that you can see the cost of surgeries. In Canada with our social healthcare system, people are not aware of the costs associated with surgeries, so when we start to see the cost of surgeries, it's going to be an eye-opener for most people as well.

There's a website in the States which acts like an auction house. If someone wants a surgery, they put in "I want knee surgery; this is my diagnosis", and surgeons can look at that and reply, "Okay, I can do that for this much." another surgeon may be able to do that fora different cost, and they can bid on it. With the medical tourism sites, most of them have their prices stated. If you pick the country you are thinking of going to and go to a site, they will tell you, "This is what the cost is." Then you should start asking questions; is that just for the surgery? What else is involved? What will the total cost be?

Unseen factors and considerations

Let's talk about your discussion to have surgery, the need for disclosure to the family and accessing the support you have. What type of types of surgery is involved and how long will it take for your body to recover. We're getting past the initial thought of doing this and looking at what factors would make you consider going abroad for surgery and what's actually involved in the process?

One of the studies I was looking at asked how people got their information about medical tourism. There were a range of stimuli; for some it was word of mouth, someone who knew someone who had had a medical procedure abroad. Or they'd looked on the internet when they were told that they needed the surgery or they wanted surgery and found medical tourism references. With others it was media, print or TV stories. Or it might be that they were familiar with another country and knew it would cost less than here.

Element Two: What Are The Unseen Factors That Are Involved When Somebody Is Considering Medical Tourism?

Disclosure to family and Doctor

WHAT WE'RE LOOKING at here is, first of all, does the doctor agree that you need this surgery? Is it a surgery that you feel you want and you have been told you can't have for some reason? Is it a cosmetic surgery or bariatric surgery? Is your doctor in agreement? It might be that your doctor has said, "You shouldn't be having this surgery because...". You might have other medical conditions that mean that this surgery is not good for you. If you are thinking of cosmetic surgery there might be something else going on and the doctor feels that the cosmetic surgery is not necessary. It might be that the anaesthetic risks or some other part of the surgical experience is going to be more detrimental to your health than the purpose of the cosmetic surgery, so your doctor might have said no. You are thinking, "No, I definitely want this, and I'm going to go and pay for it". The doctor might not be on board with that decision because of the medical considerations. It might be, yes, you need this surgery, however, before then we have to work on your weight, or your respiratory symptoms or your vascular condition, things that may affect the outcome. These might be things that need to be put in order before you are a good candidate for surgery. It may be that the doctor agrees, but for whatever reason, you are not able to have the surgery here: it could be the long wait time. Then it's up to you to decide where and when you are going to go and have the surgery.

Things to consider if you choose to circumvent your doctor's decisions and take matters into your own hands going ahead with planning to have the surgery abroad.

The biggest thing to consider is if you are going against your doctor's advice, you will need to have a doctor who is going to see you when you return after your surgery. If your doctor is saying, "No, you shouldn't be having this," you need to have a conversation with them where you can be honest and tell them; "Okay, I'm going ahead with this; are you going to support me when I come back?" The last thing you need when you return after your surgery is to try to get an appointment with your doctor, and the doctor says, "No, I don't agree with this; I'm not seeing you." Now you are stuck because you have just had surgery and need to find a doctor for your follow up appointments. It's hard enough to find a doctor when you move to a new area, however if you want to change doctors within an area and add the fact you have just had surgery abroad it's going to be even more difficult to find a doctor. A new doctor will probably not want a transfer from a local colleague and the added burden of working with case notes and test results provided from out of country.

I have heard stories about orthopaedic patients who have been told by their doctor, "No, don't go and do this," they go ahead anyway and then when they come back, their doctor won't see them and they don't have a doctor. They can't get the reference from their doctor, to be seen by another doctor, they are in this big grey area where with no healthcare support except possibly going to an Emergency department when they return. That is not the purpose of Emergency Departments so there might be a cool reception and a long wait time to be seen as emergency patients take priority.

Family in Agreement and Support

This is similar to the conversation you have with your doctor. Depending on why you are having the surgery and what surgery you are having, are you going to tell your family? Do the family agree that yes, this is a surgery you need, and are they going to support you through it? The support that you have and the mental state that you are in when you go to have surgery is a huge factor in your recovery afterward. There's lots of stress that goes along with a surgery if your family and friends are not supporting you. You are already under stress because you need the surgery for whatever reason. You are going to be doing research related to getting surgery abroad. You are going to be travelling, you are going to be in a different place that you have possibly never been to before; there's all sorts of things to take into consideration. There is a lot that happens when everyone around you is saying, "This is stupid and you are making a bad decision." It really will impact your mind set, which will affect the way the process goes for you and how you will recover from it.

You need the reassurance that the nearest and dearest to you; family, chosen family, whoever, are supporting you so that when you have a bad day or you need support, someone is going to be there to say, "Yes, that's fine; we'll help you." It's that psychological mind-set, you want this, it's something that you feel is going to change your life, you are psyched up for it, then there's someone knocking you down and putting those doubts in that will feed into your subconscious. You don't need that. You need people that say, "Yeah, it's going to be great, this is going to be good; you are going feel wonderful afterwards."

You are probably going to need somebody to travel with you for the surgery. You will have to be very selective about who goes with you as a caregiver to have the surgery. You need someone that is actually going to support you, is really going to be there for you and not just be there on holiday while you are having a surgery.

What Considerations for Work

You may already be off work due to your condition, however if you are not, one of the big considerations will be can you get the time off work to go for surgery? Are you going to be able to, take the time off work to go and get the surgery and then take the recovery time necessary afterwards? Are you going to need a graduated return to work when you return? Is your surgery multistage? Will you need any follow up after the first surgery? When will you need that surgery? Will you be able to get that time off work as well?

Then there is the money aspect. If you are not covered financially by work, do you have the money to cover your costs, including sufficient recovery time? If work doesn't cover this time away, will your job still be there when you are fit to go back?

Who Else Needs to Know and What's Really Prudent?

Advising people around you of what you are deciding to do depends on what kind of surgery you are having. You really need people on board who are going to support you. You also need all the practical things, the daily living considerations. If you are going away for an amount of time, who's going to do the day-to-day things in your home while you are away? Do you have pets that need looking after; do you have plants that need watering? Who's going to do that, so that you are not worrying about things at home when you are away?

If it comes to work, and you are going for surgery, again, depending on what the surgery is who needs to know? Why do they need to know? Is it going to help you when you come back, or is it enough for people at work to know; you are off sick and you'll be back and you'll be fine? People who you tell need to be people who are going to support you and be beneficial to your ease of mind while you are doing this and on your return to work.

It's the mundane things that need to be organized; arrangements that you want to make for grocery shopping, cooking, housekeeping, shovelling snow, gardening and things you will need help with after your surgery, you can't do it after the fact. Some of these things may have been put in place due to your current condition, it's good to consider what you will need; before, during, after surgery to aid your recovery.

Different Types of Surgery Have an Impact on the Body in Recovery

The Invasive Surgery

What does that mean? Invasive surgeries are when you

have relatively large incisions made to your body and medical instruments are used to access the area requiring the surgery. Joint replacement surgeries would be a good example of this or if you were having an "open" gastric surgery.

What does that mean? That means that the surgeon is actually going to open you up cutting through the layers of your abdomen to reach the surgical site, as opposed to when you have Minimal Invasive Surgery (MIS) where they make small incisions for access to a body cavity, or enter the body through an natural orifice with specialized instruments, they don't cut through wide layers of skin and muscle. The recovery time for these approaches is very different.

When you have an operation where you are cut through skin, fat, muscle, that's where the recovery and healing comes in; all these different layers have to heal. It doesn't matter what surgery; the fact that a wide incision was made to get there means all those layers have to heal, as well as what's be done for the surgery. That increases the possibility of complications.

As well as the consideration of the type of surgery you will be having; invasive or minimally invasive, there is also the question of which anaesthetic you will have.

If you have a general anaesthetic, it's very different than if you have a local anaesthetic or a spinal anaesthetic. There are different effects on your body. General anaesthetic can be very debilitating for your respiratory system, for your lungs, and circulation, because it stops your natural responses while they are doing the surgery.

If you are having surgery below the waist it may be decided that a spinal anaesthetic is best, the effects of the spinal anaesthetic can last 1 – 4 hours. You should have very clear instructions about when you will be allowed to sit up or get out of bed. You may be unsteady on your feet when the spinal first wears off. You'll need to make sure you ask for help when you first get out of bed after surgery. One advantage is you can normally drink fluids within an hour of the operation.

Perhaps you are going to have local anaesthetic, where it's just necessary to freeze the area that is being operated on, such as dental procedures.

There would very different things to consider with each of these anaesthetic options that would have to do with the type of surgery being performed.

General anaesthesia is a state of controlled uncon-sciousness. During a general anaesthetic, medications are used to send you to sleep, so you're unaware of sur-gery and don't move or feel pain while it's carried out.

Local anaesthesia involves numbing an area of the body using a type of medication called a local anaesthetic.

Epidural and spinal anaesthetics An epidural anaes-thetic, often referred to as an epidural, is where a local anaesthetic is continually injected through a tube into an area of the lower back called the epidural space. A spinal anaesthetic is a single injection into a similar space in the back.

Both types of anaesthetic can be used to numb large areas of the body by stopping pain signals travelling along the nerves in the spine. In some types of surgery, such as knee and hip replacements, they can be used in place of a general anaesthetic.

http://www.nhs.uk/

The Orthopaedic Surgeries

Often people who need joint surgery (hips and knees) have had reduced mobility for quite a while, before they have the surgery. Frequently this means you have put on some weight, you have not been exercising as much, so there might be things that need to be looked at prior to the surgery that will get you into the optimum state for the surgery. Maybe on some mild exercise regimen; maybe adjust the diet to lose a little weight, this would put less strain on the respiratory and circulatory system when having the surgery, so that's less adverse factors in the mix. With joint surgery, access is gained by cutting through skin, fat, muscle, bone. Then depending on the procedure, and which joint, there will cutting of bones and putting in a prosthesis. Your body will need time to adjust and it's all going to take time to heal.

There will also be physiotherapy needed after surgery. This will probably start the same day or the next day after your surgery. These are considerations that we're used to having handled by our healthcare providers, however when you go and you are getting these things a la carte, they may be considered extras and you have to make sure they are in your treatment plan.

My experience in Canada is that we don't really think about what is involved in the process. You just want the pain to stop. You are plugged into the system and you presume that the system is going to take care of you. You are going to have your surgery, they are going to tell you what to do and line up whatever you need to do afterward, and you either will or you won't conform to that plan of treatment especially concerning aftercare. I don't think there's much thought put into "what do I need to know and is this all covered?". You just assume it's going to be, because that's what we've always been taught. You get into the healthcare system here and everything gets laid out for you. This is your surgery, this is your post-surgery, these are your medications and this is your physiotherapy schedule. So if people, planning to go abroad and have surgery don't have a concept of "these are the things that are going to happen," then things could be missing that they don't think to ask about. This is a worse-case scenario, however, you don't want to go and have knee surgery and find out you are sent to the hotel next door to recover and nobody comes in to give you any physiotherapy or tells you about the exercises you need to be doing.

The Abdominal Surgeries

We talked about this in describing invasive surgeries, but what goes on here?

With abdominal surgery: if you actually do have open surgery the surgeon will open the abdominal cavity, cutting through the layers of skin, fat, and muscle to expose the viscera. This is major surgery, and again, depending on how long the procedure takes, there are many things to consider.

With all of these surgeries, there's the possibility of deep vein thrombosis. When you are having any type of surgery, especially invasive abdominal surgery, there's the possibility of DVTs. This is not usually a big consideration for the patient having surgery at home because if you are at high risk for DVTs, you will be given preventative therapy including blood thinners and calf compression legging. However, adding flying to and from a facility post-surgically will increase the DVT risk considerably.

What is DVT:

During air travel blood coagulability rises steadily and blood flow slows down, especially in the lower legs. About 3-5% of air travellers develop clots, usually painlessly, but some clots cause pain and swelling. If a clot travels to the lung it can cause pain, fainting and death. A clot in the leg is called deep vein thrombosis, DVT. A clot in the lung is pulmonary embolism, PE. Clots also form in the arterial system and in the heart, leading to heart failure and stroke.

http://www.airhealth.org/index.html

Minimally-Invasive Surgeries (MIS)

These are surgeries where two or three small incisions are made and hollow trocars, are placed to allow the surgical instruments to enter during the surgery. Surgeons use carbon dioxide gas to inflate the abdomen and move the cavity wall away from the viscera to be able to visualize the abdominal cavity. There would be a second instrument to retract (move) other organs away from the surgical site and a third instrument that would be used as the working instrument, cutting, stapling, placing bands etc.

It takes several days for the gas used to inflate the cavity to dispel in the body. That fact is something else to consider when you are thinking about flying home. The pressure of the gas in your abdomen is affected by the air pressure in the plane during the flight. Do not fly home without your surgeon's agreement.

There are occasions when minimally-invasive surgeries

have to be converted into open surgeries. A surgeon might start a procedure as minimally invasive , and then find it can't completed like that, so they have to go to an open procedure, which would be a laparotomy, or stop and not complete the procedure.

You need to have a conversation with your surgeon about this possibility prior to your surgery. What is covered in your agreement at that site? Is the site able to convert to an open surgery? Is other anaesthetic coverage available? What about post-surgery? Can they keep patients overnight at the facility? Do they have trained recovery room nurses?

You don't want to go there thinking you are going to have your gastric banding done, using a minimally invasive technique, then something happens and they find they can't do it like that, so they just close you up, and that's it. Because you still want your surgery. You want to ensure there is something in your agreement that says if they can't do it using a minimally invasive technique that they will go to an open surgery procedure. Bear in mind that if you have gone to a facility where they only perform minimally invasive surgery and something happens where they need to proceed to an open surgery, they may not have the backup at that facility for the more invasive procedure or your post-operative care.

Is there some kind of anaesthetic back up and follow through? Do they have the things in place on site in that facility in the event you need a higher level of care because of the surgery? Or are they going to have to send you somewhere else? And where is that somewhere else? How near is it? Is there an arrangement with that site to take patients from the site you have been checked into? Being the devil's advocate: what if this minimal invasive surgery goes wrong, what's the backup?

These questions shouldn't be asked just for minimal invasive surgery, they can just as reasonably be asked for any surgery; if something happens during the surgery, is there an intensive care unit, is there an anaesthetist on site, and are there staff qualified to give that extra level of care needed?

All these things happen automatically in our hospital healthcare system, where there's a backup plan and a systematic approach for all possibilities occurring in the operating room versus you having to investigate whether these contingency plans exists where you are going.

Presumably, it's all going to be fine; however it's good to have that reassurance. You want to know; if this goes wrong, where will I be going? Is it in the same facility, or somewhere else? Is it going to cost me more money? Is it factored into my agreed upon costs?

Choice of Location and reason for Choosing It

I'm in Vancouver, British Columbia where we have a very diverse ethnic community as most of us are immigrants. So, if people are looking for surgery abroad, quite often they will go to India, China or Europe. They have family there, they have the support they will need, and the costs of the procedure would probably be much less than having it done privately here. Family support, familiar language and cultural expectations, can play a large part in the decision to go abroad for surgery.

There is a lot of medical tourism in Europe these days. So when surgery is not available here or there is a long wait, people who have come here from countries such as Poland, Germany, or France, may like to go back to have their procedure. The advantage of combining an extended family visit with a surgery may also play into the decision-making. If you are going to be off work for three months, why not convalesce where you have the family ties and support.

Destination You Like, You Liked Their Website, It Looks Like a Good Place to Go

Mexico and Costa Rica are popular holiday destinations for people in Western Canada as is the Caribbean for people in Eastern Canada. This can lead people to think along the lines of; "Okay, I'm choosing this destination for my surgery because it's somewhere that I've been and I like", or "I want to go to that country and they offer medical tourism."

There are so many countries and areas these days that have some aspect of medical tourism happening.

Speciality, Expertise, and Reputation

There are also locations that specialize in particular surgeries and people may make decisions regarding location based on the level of specialty available.

In Canada we have "Snowbirds" retirees who travel south for the winter heading for the warmer weather. From Vancouver a lot of the Snowbirds head to Arizona or Mexico. While they are away for the winter, conversations often turn to various dental procedures they might need and the related costs. After chatting with fellow travellers many people are finding themselves in the town of Los Algodones near Yuma, a former farm town that now claims to be the "dental centre of Mexico." In fact I'm told you can park your car in Yuma, walk across the border, and you'll find about 70 dentists in town! You can have your dental procedure, walk back, and then go and have a margarita in the evening to celebrate the money you saved. It's estimated that roughly 6,000 to 12,000 Canadians travel to Mexico, including Los Algodones, for dental care every year usually between October and April.

> I read one story of a man who went to a clinic in Los Algodones; he went in their winter. He had his pick of dentists: The one he chose was on a block with nine clinics. He bought a set of dentures for a considerably reduced cost. "I haven't been to a dentist in Canada for 50 years," he said, noting: "I haven't had any teeth for 50 years either."

In Europe, Italy and Poland are known for providing the liberation procedure". This procedure was developed in Italy by a surgeon who found it to be beneficial to people with Multiple Sclerosis (MS). Chronic Cerebrospinal Venous Insufficiency (CCSVI) is a narrowing of veins in the neck and chest that carry blood away from the brain and spinal cord. The treatment for CCSVI is called endovascular surgery, "liberation therapy", or the "liberation procedure." It involves placing a tiny balloon or tube called a stent inside a blocked vein in the neck to open it and restore blood flow out of the brain and spinal cord. Researchers have been studying whether treating CCSVI by opening up blocked veins can improve symptoms of MS. In Canada it is still listed as an experimental procedure for people with MS so is not covered by Healthcare.

Brazil is the number one country for plastic surgery, closely followed by Thailand. Thailand has a huge medical tourism industry. One of the most reputable hospitals there treats 520,000 international patients a year from 190 countries. Most of their doctors do post-graduate training overseas and the facility offers all surgical specialities.

India is marketing itself as one of the top three destinations in Asia for medical tourists, stating it is *"known mostly for its cost-effective medical treatments along with high standards in cardiology, orthopaedics, nephrology, oncology and neuro surgery"* (Times of India Sept 1st 2014)

When considering surgery abroad, it will depend on where you want to go, what speciality you need and what you are looking for in terms of destination. It may look like a nice destination to visit, however, it might not be the best country or facility for the type of surgery you are considering and vice-versa. You might be considering somewhere where they are specialists in your surgery, however there's going to be a lot of travel. For example, travelling to Thailand is definitely a much longer proposition than to Mexico from Vancouver. The length of travel pre and post-surgery should be a large factor when deciding where to have your surgery.

Price and the Convenience

Medical tourism websites usually show their comparative costs in American dollars. The rule of thumb seems to be when looking at India and Thailand, that surgeries in these countries can be less than a quarter of what you would pay here, including the cost of travel, and the hotel for you and your caregiver. Therefore, you are looking at a huge reduction of costs. For dental surgery in Mexico, you might look at a procedure here that's $3,000, and see the same procedure advertised for $500 there. With these advertised price differences it's easy to see why people are pursuing surgery abroad.

However, when you are looking at the price difference, you really have to look at the quality, not the quantity. I used the example of getting a car repaired earlier in the book. If you have a problem with the repair you can go back to the garage and ask them to fix it. In that case you'd want a garage nearby to get back to conveniently, one that used the original manufactures parts. With any surgery your body is a limited resource, once something has been removed or altered there's less to work with if anything else goes wrong. You need to know you can go back to the surgeon as soon as a problem arises as it will only get more complicated the longer it's left.

Convenience factors that needs to be considered

How far you travel for your surgery; how long you will need to recovery post-surgery time, and how convenient is it to travel to the facility.

You don't want to be travelling for a surgery where you have to make three plane changes and it's going to take a day or two to get there. You may be okay with this long travel schedule when you go to the facility. However when you come back, you are post-surgery, so that all will not only add to the time you have to be in transit, but it may also have a detrimental effect to your recovery.

For example, the air pressure in the plane can be detrimental to any kind of gastric surgery. It is essential to ensure that you have had enough recovery post-surgery before you are flying. You must check with your surgeon and ask "Is it okay for me to fly now?" You don't want anything happening on the plane.

With joint surgery, for your hip or your knee, you don't want to be travelling and sitting on a plane for days on end, not being able to move. With normal air travel there is the risk of deep vein thromboses (DVTs) caused by sitting for long periods in a cramped position, this is considerably increased after surgery.

> During air travel blood coagulability rises steadily and blood flow slows down, especially in the lower legs. About 3-5% of air travellers develop clots, usually painlessly, but some clots cause pain and swelling. If a clot travels to the lung it can cause pain, fainting and death. A clot in the leg is called deep vein thrombosis, DVT. A clot in the lung is pulmonary embolism, PE. Clots also form in the arterial system and in the heart, leading to heart failure and stroke.
>
> http://www.airhealth.org/index.html

There is also the possibility that your immune system will be slightly compromised due to the surgery. We all know that travelling on the plane; you are more likely to be susceptible to getting sick because of the crowded conditions, the recirculated air and the confined space. If you have had a general anaesthetic your respiratory system is probably functioning slightly less than what it would. Being on a plane and having someone sitting next to you hacking and coughing for twelve hours is not going to do you any good.

It's absolutely essential that you get the final sign off from your surgeon before you travel home.

Follow up after surgery

Sometimes you can't tell if the surgery was totally successful for a while afterward. How can you get the follow-up you require once you return to your home country?

For example, who would be doing the follow-up and

possible repair if your teeth don't line up and you can't chew properly, but you can't tell because there was swelling after your surgery? If you need to have the alignment checked once the swelling subsides, it could be pricey if you have already left the country.

With bariatric gastric band surgery, the band has to be tightened or adjusted post-surgery. Who's going to do that follow up procedure? Is there someone near your home who's going to do it? Is there some kind of liaison between the foreign facility and your home town doctor for follow- up, or do you have to go back to the facility abroad?

Things you have to think of in terms of the cost to yourself, not just the price tag on the website.

You definitely have to research the overall costs and the timeframe. If you are having something done that needs a follow up in six months or a year, is the package that you are paying for including that, or is it a separate package, and how much will that be in the long term for the full course of treatment?

The Timeframe, Ease of Travel and Length of Stay Necessary for a Safe Return.

Economics vs. Logistics

Is it an easy country to travel to? Do you need to have medical vaccinations and visas to get into the country?

Before going anywhere abroad as a regular traveller, you will need to check if you require a visa or a series of vaccinations, and ensure you have travel insurance. If you are going to be a medical tourist, you have to make sure that you have the right kind of health and travel insurance. You can't assume that a regular travel health insurance will cover you if you have surgery, especially if something goes wrong because of the surgery and you need to be airlifted back home. You really have to look into whether the health insurance you get for the travel will cover your surgery as well.

With the visa, it's not just for you; it's also for whoever's accompanying you, and will there be any different visa requirements necessary because you are going into surgery? Does that affect things? Are there any different vaccinations you need, or are the vaccinations that you are told you need to go to the country detrimental to the surgery that you are going to have while there? It might interact with something that they want to give you, or there might be some fine print that says, "Don't take blood thinners," or "don't take X, until X months after this vaccination." Who do you ask? How will you know this?

You should be discussing this fully with your regular doctor who's supporting you prior to the travel for surgery or with your surgeon at the facility where you are going. Do you need vaccinations? Will they be detrimental to the surgery you are going to have abroad?

Factor in Recovery Time and Safety in Planning your Trip

When discussing your surgery with staff at the facility you have chosen you should be asking how long after surgery to wait before you travel. If you are going to have a surgery and you will be in hospital for three days and then need at least fourteen days afterwards before you travel, how will that be arranged? Is this included in the package that they are selling you? Do they provide convalescence somewhere away from the hospital?

On one of the websites I was looking at, if someone went for hip surgery, they factored in X number of days at the hospital and then they sent them to a partnership resort for the convalescence. The resort worked with the hospital, so was accustomed to catering to post surgery clients. That situation was great. One of the other sites I was looking at dealt with physiotherapy; they had a plan custom made for each of their clients for exactly when and what treatment should occur. The example I saw was actually a teenager; he had shoulder surgery, and prior to going home, there was a discussion between the foreign facility physiotherapist and the physiotherapist he would be seeing when he returned home outlining the whole physiotherapy plan. "This is what needs to happen for your physical therapy when you get home, and we'll be liaising with that physical therapist to make sure that you are on track."

Language Familiarity and Cultural Comfort

If you are considering going to another country; do you speak the language, or are there people in that facility who speak your language? I've been talking about the big hospitals in medical tourism, however a lot of people will probably be going to small clinics, especially for dental treatments or plastic surgeries.

If you are having dental procedures, you are probably going to a dental office. Does that dental office have staff who speak English? Are they going to speak English to a level where they understand when you are in pain or have a problem? If you are going for plastic surgery, same thing: it might not be a big facility, it might just be a small clinic.

Quite often they might be a clinic with one operating room. You will have a consultation with the surgeon in the clinic, your surgery in their operating room, then, post-surgery you will probably stay in a hotel nearby You need to know how this arrangement works. If something happens to you on the post-surgery night, who do you call? How do you call them; via the hotel phone or do you have a direct dial cell phone? Do you know the person you will be speaking to, have they been introduced to you, do they understand you? Will they be able to check your dressing or increase your pain medication if needed?

You should also be asking about the reports you will need to bring back with you describing your surgery, medications given, and follow up antibiotics or therapy required. It's essential that these reports be in your language, so that when you get home your healthcare provider can access the information as soon as possible. The reports should include surgical procedure, medications, x-rays, blood tests etc. that you have when you are abroad.

These reports must come back *with* you because you need to be checking in with your healthcare practioner as soon as you come back. (You will have made the appointment before you left the country to have the surgery.) The reports may be hand written, but must be legible; they will most likely be either on a CD or USB. Ask to see these files on a computer screen to ensure they can be read in whatever format you are given.

Travel Companion

Your choice of travel companion is something I really have to emphasize. You must be very careful who you decide take with you. The person may be someone who's a great buddy or a partner, but might be really useless in a hospital situation. They may not be a good traveller, and end up getting sick, which would result in you being worried about them and they wouldn't be able to concentrate on your recovery.

It might be that the person you choose hasn't travelled and when you arrive they have a problem adapting to another culture. Whoever goes with you has to be your advocate and to have you as their number one priority. They cannot think they are just going for a holiday. It must be someone who can make sure that when you can't talk because you are post-surgery, your basic needs are going to be looked after. Ensuring you are comfortable, you have adequate pain relief, you have enough to drink and that you can use the washroom. They have to be there as your advocate, not just your buddy on a holiday.

The Support and Ease of the Process and the Ability to Get Follow Up

Follow Up at Home to Provide Continuity of Care?

Before you set off for surgery abroad you should know if your doctor going to support your plan and that are they are willing to support you when you come back. You need to have a discussion with your doctor prior to the surgery because their decision to support you post-surgery will depend on the type of surgery you are planning to have, and if your doctor is in agreement for you to have that particular surgery.

If they are not supportive, then who will be your medical practioner when you get back? You should arrange this before you go, because when you come back after surgery is not the time to start making phone calls, or turning up at offices trying to get doctors to see you. It's all going to add to your stress and won't help in your recovery. You need to make sure that you have the medical support, whether, for example a doctor; physiotherapy, nutritionist, or dietary support. Do you know which medications you will need? Are you going to be on a course of antibiotics? Do you have to take them prior to surgery or have them with you so you can start immediately after the surgery? How long do you have to take them? Who's going to prescribe medications when you come back if necessary? Can it be prescribed before you go?

The Time Off, Support, Rehab, and Medications for a Complete Recovery

Have you made these arrangements or considered this?

If you have ever tried to get appointments with healthcare practioners, you'll know that there is always a waiting period, especially if you are a new patient. You might have to wait weeks or a month to get an appointment. Therefore, before your surgery, you will need to make sure that you have booked your appointment with the physiotherapist or whomever you need to follow-up with when you come back. Also, check if you need repeat blood tests, X-rays, medication and how often you need to go to physio. Confirm what else might be needed as a follow-up.

Documentation of your procedure, what kind of documentation is necessary?

The documentation about your procedure has to be in the right language for follow up when you arrive home.

You will need a complete report of your surgery including, the anaesthetic and any medications given while you are away. This is necessary so that when you come back, your doctor has a complete overview of what happened to you. "I went and had this surgery. Here is the report with the anaesthetic information; these are the drugs that were given, these are the drugs that I've come back on (you might be on antibiotics); here's the x-ray report and current blood tests." This gives your doctor a complete overview of everything that happened to you and what you were taking while you were there and since your return. So then they know how to step in and continue that care.

What kinds of problems would there be if this information was incomplete or in another language?

In both cases the doctor has to rely on what you are telling them has happened to you while you have been away. Most people when they are in meetings with doctors catch one in three words of what the doctor's telling them has happened. (It's similar to an increase in the patients' blood pressure in White Coat Syndrome) and they don't know exactly what's happened. Bearing this in mind, a written message that a healthcare provider can actually read is crucial: "On this date, this is the surgery that actually happened. We did this, this, and this." If you need help with a medical problem and this report is written in another language, or is illegible, it will take time to get a translation or new, legible copy. Time you should be being treated for your health issue.

There's also the risk of contraindication for certain medications. Unless your doctor knows exactly which medication you have received (or are still taking) they will not be able to take the required precautions if something happens. This can be quite dangerous.

I've often seen articles on the use of generic drugs as opposed to Brand Named products. These "knock-off" drugs are manufactured for a fraction of the price, (cutting down on the costs for a clinic) as long as the generic products are perfect replicas there is no problem for the consumer. The problems start when these drugs have different active ingredients that are absorbed into the blood stream differently or there is a change in the in-active ingredients; binders, fillers and dyes. If you are having a reaction to a drug it maybe that you were given a generic drug and you are reacting to these changed ingredients.

If you are on a course of antibiotics post -surgery, how are you instructed to be taking it? What happens if you don't complete the full course or if you react to the antibiotics you are given? If these problems don't show up until you reach home your doctor will need to know exactly which drug you have been given to be able to change or adapt the dosage.

Requirement to Follow Up Surgery or Other Procedures

Surgeries are usually followed up at least a month or six week afterwards to see how patients are doing after their surgery. The healthcare professional wants to ensure there's no infection and to see how the scar is healing. There should be someone looking at you at least six weeks afterward surgery to say, "Yes, this is healing fine; yes, this is doing great." That is the minimum you should arrange.

A procedure like a gastric band will need to be followed up to see if the band needs to be tightened or loosened, depending on what's happening with your change in eating habits. There may also be a follow-up in six months or a year for an adjustment, as you lose weight and change your eating habits.

Element Three: Evaluation Of The Best And Safest Option

Logistics: Scheduling Everything

THERE ARE SEVERAL things to consider when you are going to have surgery. The primary consideration is to have an idea of the timeframe of the surgery and recovery period. You should not be thinking along the lines of a vacation. "Okay, I'm going to have two weeks' vacation, I'm going to come back, and it's all going to be perfect." This is very different from going on vacation; this is surgery abroad. A surgical experience at home can be traumatic enough because it's out of most people's usual experience, (apart from seeing some hospital dramas on TV and in films). Now you are planning for surgery and in addition have to consider the actual time this is going to take out of your life, as well as everything that will be affected by it.

Will you need to be away for two weeks? What preparation is there before the surgery; exercise, diet to optimum weight, stop smoking? What is the overall recovery time needed? How long is the convalescence afterwards? Is a gradual return to work required? How much physiotherapy will be needed? Will you need dietary counselling or to join a support group? All these factors and more need to be considered in this big picture of your surgery and their effects on the timeframe.

You may have been told that the surgery only takes X number of hours and you need X many days at the facility or nearby before going home. However, you also have to consider where will you are doing the majority of your recovery, how much time you will need off work and what will need to be in place during that time.

It's very different if someone were having cosmetic surgery (for example, a nose or chin reshaping). The surgery's not going to take long. However, you have to recover for weeks afterward, as you wait for the bruising to go down, especially if you don't want people to know you have had it done. So how long will it actually take? If you are having orthopaedic surgery, say a hip or knee replacement how long is it going to take before you can walk a distance without crutches, and ease back into the normal daily activities we all take for granted? Depending on the surgery, there will be very different timeframes.

If you have bariatric surgery, the surgery itself might only be as a day patient if you have a gastric band, however, you have to factor in time before the surgery where you are working to get into optimal health. Afterward, there are a lot of things to do with your diet, exercise and mental wellbeing. Physically, it's not that it's invasive a surgery, however there are huge changes in your metabolism and diet that might affect work, and travel. There is also the emotional roller coaster; the weight doesn't disappear with the surgery, so finding a support group of patients who have had the procedure and know what it's like will be important for you. These are not necessarily in-person groups, they may be Chat Rooms or Skype calls. Find out about what's available before your surgery so you can participate as soon as you return home.

Making the Arrangements to Get the Time off Work.

Actually creating that space and time in your life, what are the factors do you need to consider?

Is the surgery you are proposing something that's seen as a requirement and can you get the paid sick leave? Is it cosmetic surgery you don't want work to know about? Will your employer still give you the time off? Will it be paid leave from work, or will it be something where you'll have to take a leave of absence and pay for yourself? This will be something else to factor into the cost of the surgery, travel and the convalescence; you might not be earning anything. Have you got the flexibility for these financial considerations?

How do you get a doctor's note for work?

I spoke of having the support of your doctor for the surgery you are planning. If the paid sick time off work is dependent on a doctor's note stating you will be off due to surgery, and if your regular doctor is not supporting the surgery you are planning, who is going to write that note for you? Will it be accepted by your employers? Will it be covered by their health plan? You need to be aware if there is some small print in your benefits package that states only your regular doctor or a doctor you are referred to by the health plan can sign the note regarding the need for you to have elective surgery.

Not having the backing of a healthcare plan provided by your employer may greatly increase the costs of surgery abroad.

Financial Considerations and the Feasibility of Going Ahead with This

Because of Canada's healthcare system, employees expect that their employer will cover their sick leave, convalescence recovery and gradual return to work, if needed. While they are in the hospital, everything is covered, including doctors, nurses, respiratory therapy, drugs and food. Patients will probably receive physical therapy while in hospital and a set number of visits to the hospital physiotherapy department after they are discharged. The cost of these outpatient visits will probably be covered as well. It's these things that we take for granted at home. However, when it comes to arranging your surgery package abroad you really have to consider the cost of all aspects. This is your choice; you are paying for it all.

Caregivers and Timing, Time Off.

As well as having time off to get the surgery, most people will take someone with them when they travel abroad for surgery; someone to be their caregiver, the support while they are away. It might be a partner, best friend or a relative, now you have to consider how they will get the time off work. Are you going to pay them and their expenses? How's that going to work out? How much time do you actually need to have them with you? Is it just while you are abroad? Do you need someone to stay with you when you are at home afterward? How are you going to cover those costs? Will you need nursing support when you get home? Is your caregiver able to give you that?

You will need to have healthcare appointments when you come back.

When you return, you'll need a follow up appointment with your doctor (or another doctor if your doctor won't see you regarding the surgery). You'll also need physiotherapy if you are having orthopaedic surgery. There's usually a time lag to get these appointments, so you should be planning the appointments before you go. You must ensure you have a doctor and physiotherapists who are going to support you when you come back. We discussed this earlier. Does your doctor or physiotherapist agree with you going abroad to have this done and are they willing to see you when you return? If they are not, who are you going to see? You'll probably need to start your physiotherapy within days of coming back, so you'll have to have a physiotherapist pre-booked. A doctor also has to see you when you come back to follow-up. You need to know which doctor you are going to see and make sure that you have an appointment to see them within six weeks of having the surgery. You should definitely see a surgeon or doctor to check that you are doing okay in the initial recovery stage. All of that needs to all be arranged before you go.

Making the Arrangements for Travel & the Procedures

Using facilitators or doing it yourself.

Surgery is a huge step into the unknown for most people. It might be something that is like a carrot dangling in front of you; it's perceived as the thing that is going to change your life. However, do you actually know what's involved? Most people's experience of surgery is what they see on TV or in films. It's not really like that; that's the media version of it. There's lots of things going on in the background that make up the whole experience, that contribute to the safe and smooth running of the process, and if you add into that travelling abroad for surgery, things expand exponentially.

For example, there are many details in just planning a holiday abroad. You are looking for the best flight, the best hotel, whether it is it all-inclusive or not, and how you get there from the airport. If you add into the mix, "Okay, what hospital am I going to? Who's the surgeon? How do I get there? How do I talk to them? How long is it going to take? What happens after the surgery? Do I go directly to the hospital, or do I go to the hotel, then the hospital? Where do I go after the surgery?" If you add all of that into it, the question becomes, do you actually want to be doing everything yourself, adding to your stress level before you go have surgery, or do you want to find a professional who arranges surgery abroad for clients?

There are people out there who are called Medical Tourism Facilitators. They are basically like a travel agent who specializes in arranging surgery abroad for clients. Many of the medical tourism facilitators have certifications, for tourism and with medical tourism associations. They will quite often be linked to a facility in the country that they specialize in, or are perhaps an independent broker able to advise you on the country of your choice. They will arrange everything like an all-inclusive holiday; however it will be an all-inclusive package for your travel *and* surgery. You have to decide if you are comfortable making all the arrangements yourself or if you'd like someone to arrange it all for you.

Comparison Shopping: What Are You Getting?

Most people's initial contact with medical tourism is online. You want a particular surgery or may need it in the future and have heard about surgery abroad being less expensive. The initial search may be a subject search for the type of surgery, then it can be narrowed down to a country that you think you'd like to go to, or the country you are from. After that, you'll probably pick three or four facilities, and then make a decision usually based on price. There can be lots of hidden costs if you don't ask the right questions. You don't necessarily know what you are getting. Most people won't know which questions to ask.

It's very hard to shop based on the price you see on the site.

When you are looking for a facility abroad to have your surgery, you will find that many websites quote prices after you fill in a short questionnaire about the surgery you require. There's the price you see on the site, however you also have to ask, "Is this the total price; is there anything else I'll have to pay for?" You don't want to be in a foreign country having had surgery and then, before you can leave, you are told there's X hundred dollars extra that you have to pay. That's why it can be quite prudent to hire someone like a medical tourism facilitator who knows where these hidden costs can lie.

Choosing a Facilitator, what factors are there to consider?

As with all service industry providers someone might put up their shingle as a medical tourism facilitator; however you will want to be assured of their background and their experience before you commit to employing them to facilitate your surgery. The range of people calling themselves medical tourism facilitators is as broad as the topic of surgery itself. There may be someone who has arranged a surgery for friends or family in their mutual country of origin. Inspired by a successful outcome they may think, "That went well I could start a business doing it". Ideally you need someone who's actually taken a course and knows about the medical tourism industry. They should have some medical training or background. Some questions to consider are: Do they have travel agent or tourism experience? Do they openly identify if they are affiliated with the facility they are recommending to you, or do they provide an independent search based on what you need? There can be all sorts of people with varying levels of expertise out there in the mix. I've read about one man who was a truck driver and he thought it would be a good to get into this business as he travelled around a lot. His business didn't last very long.

Are you going to ask the truck driver to arrange your surgery? It's a bit like asking the surgeon to deliver your sofa. You need to ask someone who's got a medical background and who knows the travel and tourism industry. You really have to ask them important questions such as, what their training is; how long they have been medical tourism facilitators. It is also imperative to ask them to provide references from people who they've dealt with, so you can contact past clients to ensure that they provide a good service.

 How to interview your facilitator and criteria
Go to areusafe.ca to download the checklist

How much is that going to cost you? As the client do you pay them, or are they being paid a commission by the facilities they are dealing with? Are they possibly being paid by both you and the facility? Does that matter?

How Much Do You Want Everything Handled for You and What Can You Deal with Yourself?

Maybe there's a balance between what you can do as far as research and what a medical tourism facilitator can complete for you regarding the details.

It might be that you can do some searching around online and you might decide, "Okay, I've got this, and I really want to go to Mexico, because that's only four hours away and I feel comfortable with that." Or, "I don't like flying; I could drive there." Mode of travel might be another consideration that comes into your decision . Some people are comfortable using the Internet and they can do a lot of the research themselves, but they might not feel so comfortable with having a conversation with the staff or surgeon of the facility. It's out of their comfort zone. You have to know what you are comfortable with and what you are capable of doing when it comes to organizing surgery abroad. Are you okay when you book your own holidays? Do you always turn up at great places and everything's fine? Or do you have some real slips in judgement when you pick something that was a great price but when you arrive it's not finished being built yet or is located in a much less desirable area that you expected?

How Do You Make the Best Choice of the Safest & Best Facility?

Researching the Facility by Yourself

When you are researching on the internet you have got to be very careful, because anybody can put up an absolutely amazing looking website, (think of the scam emails with sites that look like banks or credit card companies). You really have to do your due diligence and make sure you follow up on all information provided. An easy test is to make a phone call to the website contact to check that somebody picks up the phone and can actually speak English or French or whatever language they promise. It's a very good start if the phone number on their website is answered in person, not a machine, and gets you to someone who understands you straight away. If the facility doesn't have the attention to detail where the person on the phone can understand you that's not a good indication of the communication skills for the facility, especially when you are vulnerable after surgery.

Get Support in Finding the Best and Safest Option for Your Specific Situation

A lot of people use the Internet to join groups that reflect their different problems. People with joint problems, with weight and with low esteem issues can belong to groups and chat rooms on the Internet and have circles of friends who have similar conditions. Within those friends, you might find someone who has already had surgery abroad, or who knows someone that's done it. These social groups are great places to ask for advice such as, "Do you know somebody who's done this? Where did they go? How did they choose? Did they do it themselves or did they use a facilitator? Who did they use?"

When you are interviewing medical facilitators, ask them direct questions like, "Can you put me in contact with someone you've helped in a similar situation so I can ask about their experience?" Check if the facilitator has been to the healthcare facility recently and why they are recommending it. Get as much information as you can to find out what it is about that facility's option that is best for your specific situation.

Interviewing the Facility Doctors and Getting the Answers You Need

"Do I have to do this on top of having someone choose the facility for me?"

I would make sure that if someone is providing medical tourism facilitator services for you, that you feel very comfortable in their level of medical expertise and that they have actually done due diligence regarding your surgery. You should speak to people who have dealt with them before and know that past clients feel comfortable recommending their service and the facility suggested for you. The medical tourism facilitator you choose should be able to provide you will all the answers regarding the surgeon and staff qualifications at the site, their expertise with your particular surgery and details about the standards adhered to by the facility. Your contact with the facility and surgeon will be related to your pre-surgery consultation. This may be a phone call, Skype or a webinar connection.

 Questions you should be asking about the facility, checklist available on <u>areusafe.ca</u> to download.

Do You Have Support from the Facility after the Fact?

There are certain types of surgical procedures that need to have scheduled follow up, like that needed with a gastric band. The band will need to be tightened or loosened after the surgery, so who does that? Do you have to go back in six weeks or a year? Does the facility have some arrangement with a doctor in your locale that you can go to and they will do it? What happens if something goes wrong with a surgery that you have abroad, such as a surgical site infection? Do you go back to that facility, or stay local, and go to emergency? Who deals with it? What is the contact you have with the facility after the fact? Is there follow up built in to your contract with them and for how long?

I've heard that for some facilities abroad, the surgeon or a member of the medical staff from the facility will phone up after you have returned home to see how you are doing. As part of their service some of the medical tourism facilitators' offer that they'll meet you at the airport when you come home, to make sure you have arrived safely. Some medical tourism facilitators who specialize in clients, who have had bariatric surgery, offer support groups for clients after surgery.

With bariatric surgery it's not just about having the surgery, it's maintaining the momentum afterward. A lot of it is the psychological reinforcement; this is how life is going to be, by following this regime you will succeed in your desired weight loss and by relying on a support group of peers who have been through the same experience to help you through it.

Money: Do You Have Money Set Aside For This Surgery, And Then Some, As a Safety Net?

The cost of surgery abroad is not just the surgery, it's all the incidentals. I mentioned previously that there will be time off work (paid or unpaid), medications, the surgery itself, the travel and the cost of your companion. There's also follow up costs like the physiotherapy, continued medications, or dietary requirements. Do you have the money to cover all these costs? Do you have a contingency plan and money to follow through if there are problems with your recovery time and it has to be extended or if you have to return to the facility where you had your surgery?

What Are the True Costs When Adding It All Up?

When you are looking on the website, you might see the cost of surgery stated and you think:, "Okay, I'm going to have this surgery, it would to cost me $40,000 here and it's going to cost me $6,000 there, so great, look at the money that I've saved." Often that's just the cost of the surgery. You have to look at all costs and not get swept away with, "Oh, it's only going to cost me $6,000." It's all those other incidentals that might round it up and you might end up with a bill for $12,000. So you can get caught out by thinking, "I've got an $8,000 nest egg; I can do this." And then it's a $12,000 expense, how are you going to cover that?

 Checklist of cost factors to consider areusafe.ca to download

Contingency Funds, What do you need in contingency?

This is the same thing we're all told by financial planners: *you should have at least three months' worth of money in case you lose your job*. It's the same thing with having surgery abroad: you should have money so that if something does goes wrong and there are some added costs, added time off work that you have the emergency funds to actually pay for that unexpected extension of time when you won't be working. Another thing to consider is the person who's going with you as your caregiver; something might happen to them as a traveller. Do you cover their costs? That's part of the contingency planning as well. What happens if they have an accident while they are away and they need surgery, or they catch a bug and they are off work when they come back? Are you going to have to cover them financially? Don't forget when you are planning that the minimum financial buffer needs to include your caregiver.

Your travel companions health:

A study of 247 patients in a Calgary Health Region in Canada with multi-drug resistant E.coli determined that 72% of the infections were acquired in the community rather than in a hospital setting and that international travel was a "major risk factor" associated with developing the infection.

Unseen Travelers: Medical Tourism and the Spread of Infectious Disease.

Jill R Hodges and Ann Marie Kimball (2012)

Another thing to factor in is insurance costs.

The insurance you require for surgery abroad is not going to be regular traveller's insurance. You have to be upfront when buying the insurance and say that you are going abroad for a particular type of surgery, because if you don't get the right insurance, and something happens where you need to make a claim, the insurance company is not going to pay out. Say you need to come back due to a medical emergency, you need a medivac evacuation, or something happens to your caregiver and they need to come back: how smoothly this goes will all depend on the right travel and health insurance you purchase. You have to make sure that you have got the right insurance and be very honest with the insurance broker about why you are going abroad. The bottom line is you need to make sure that the coverage you have will actually pay out if something goes wrong for you and your caregiver.

I noticed when I last renewed my travel insurance for the year that the policy had been updated to have an exclusion clause for medical procedures done abroad. Insurance companies are much more aware of medical tourism and the problems that can occur with surgeries abroad than the majority of the general population.

When you buy regular holiday travel insurance it often has a medivac option where the insurance company will pay to have you transported home. This is excluded if you have gone for elective surgery, as it's not an accident or emergency while on vacation.

In addition when you are flying, you have to tell the airline that you have had surgery. Airlines have contingency plans and risk management plans that come into play when there's someone on the plane who has a potential health problem, or a medical emergency while on the plane. All airlines carry a

basic emergency kit and will ask for assistance from any doctors on the plane if the need arises. I also understand there are
doctors on call for airlines. The doctor will be made aware of
passengers who have potential medical conditions and which
flights they are on. If the airlines don't know you have had
surgery and there is a medical emergency they will be unable
to get you the help you need in the most timely manner.

Your Companion, Support, and Spokesperson Who Can Assess Your Ability Post Surgery

Agreement with the Companion of the Level of Support They Will Provide

It is essential that you can communicate easily with the
person who accompanies you abroad for your surgery. They
really have to know you because they are going to be the person who is looking out for you, and advocating for you in a
foreign country. You have to be able to talk to this person on
a very intimate level. You must ensure it's somebody you can
talk to about intimate bodily functions because post-surgery,
the best questions after all surgery are, "Can you pass urine?"
and "Have you had your bowels open today?" You have got
to have someone who's willing to be an active intermediary
between you and the nursing staff. Would you be comfortable discussing bodily functions with the next-door neigh-
bour who's come with you as your caregiver? You have to be
comfortable with and confident in the level of support they
can give you.

The Ability of Your Companion to Act as a Spokesperson

When choosing who accompanies you as your care giver make sure they are comfortable in a hospital settings and speaking to medical staff. Some people are really great and very engaged in life, but you walk them into a hospital and they close right down. They just can't function in a hospital. It's just totally out of their realm, and the person who you know who would normally support you in anything suddenly, when they are in the hospital, will just sit there. Basically you have to make sure that the companion who accompanies you is able to function in that potentially stressful situation, for both you and for them. It will be a different country, possibly a different language they will be responsible for someone who's had surgery and is not capable of looking after themselves for X number of hours post-surgery. Are they going to be able to step up to the plate and say, "It looks like she's in pain," or, "Can she have some water?" "It's hot; can we get a fan in here?" Will they be able to do this? Is this person able to look out for you, to be the intermediary and advocate that you need?

The caregivers are also going to have some decision-making capacity should something arise; do they know your exact wishes?

If something happens and a decision needs to be made, and you can't communicate, your caregiver needs to be able to make that decision. If you are out of commission and the facility needs consent to go-ahead on something more than you originally signed for, can this caregiver say; "Yes, do it"?

Check that this is covered in the consent form you sign; they may have a clause: "*and/or related procedures*". Whereby if the surgeon found an abnormality during the procedure requiring another surgery, they might just proceed with that surgery and you could be facing a much higher surgical cost.

The Ability of This Person to Communicate on the Most Basic Level of Your Needs, Pain, and Comfort

The person, who accompanies you, can't be someone for whom you always have to put on a brave face and tough it out. It has to be someone who can see that the pain medication is not working or you are not comfortable. They have to be aware that the facility keeps giving you orange juice and you hate orange juice but you like apple juice. You want someone there who knows you, can anticipate your needs, has attention to detail and is willing and able to help you. It will reduce your stress and aid your recovery.

The Physical Ability to Handle Travel, Caregiving, Exertion, and Emotional Stress

In this section I have to ask you, are you a good traveller? Some people don't travel well, some people don't fly well. Some people might choose a medical tourism facility that they can drive, or travel by train because they don't like flying. Do you need time to recover from a flight? Do you know that it takes you a day or so once you have flown to actually settle down physically? You need to build all that in to your plans and it will be the same with your caregiver. Are they good travellers or not?

When you arrive, are you going to plan to do some kind of tourism things beforehand? Have you spoken to your surgeon about this, because you don't want to be dashing around up and down volcanoes or exploring the rain forest if you are supposed to be resting before the surgery. You also don't want to expose yourself or your care giver to any type of local hazards prior to the surgery. This may be a simple as not being a tourist before the surgery and only eating at the hotel or healthcare facility. There is a lot of emotional stress associated with travelling. Where are you going? What's it going to be like? These anxieties, including the anticipation around the surgery, all builds into your pre-operative stress level. You can be fairly stressed out when you arrive at your destination.

Information is the key. The more you know, the more prepared you can be, and this is not the time to be an ostrich and stick your head in the sand.

You want to know as much as possible, then you are prepared for hopefully every eventuality, rather than things coming as a surprise. The smoother it is, the fewer surprises, the better off you will be when you have had your surgery. You'll be calmer and more relaxed and aware of the whole process.

Element Four: Getting It Done: Following Through On the Plans

Consultation with the surgeon, bloodwork and tests, pre-surgery timing, ensuring it gets done, or is it a no-go from here?

Once you have decided that you are definitely going to have your surgery abroad and have researched the country and facilities that provide the surgery you want via their websites, you'll want to have a conversation either with someone at the facility or the medical tourism facilitator. Then you need a consultation with your surgeon, or at least the intake nurse at the facility. Quite often on these websites, they'll arrange a phone call or a Skype conversation where you actually see and talk to a person at the site. So instead of going to the doctor's office, you are Skyping the consultation. Sometimes the medical tourism facilitator might go through a questionnaire with you and send it to the facility before the call so they have the bulk of your information in front of them for the call. However, I find that more often there is some actual contact by phone and Skype, usually with the surgeon.

Talking to the surgeon

I think that you should be speaking directly with the surgeon before you leave the country. You want to know that you can communicate easily with the surgeon and at least have a look at the surgeon before you go there. Sometimes the facilitator will have completed a questionnaire with you prior to the call that keeps the conversation on track and shortens the online consultation.

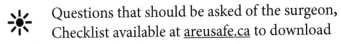 Questions that should be asked of the surgeon, Checklist available at areusafe.ca to download

I've provided a checklist of questions for you to ask the surgeon because I know a lot of people's minds go blank when they are sitting in front of someone with a white coat. You forget every third word that you were going to ask or even what they say. So the checklist is to keep you on track and give you something to refer to after the call. You may even think of recording the call; most cell phones have the capacity to record these days.

Pre-surgery tests or procedures that may need to be done prior to you travelling abroad.

Depending on which surgery you are having, there's obviously going to be some things that you need to do beforehand to get ready. You are probably going to have blood tests and x-rays. There should be some kind of anesthetic evaluation, or at least a questionnaire about what your heart and lungs are like before you are going to have this surgery. You might need to be doing some physical exercises, or it's might be exercises to get you into the practice of deep breathing to help you inflate your lungs as much as possible to remove all traces of the anaesthetic gases post-surgery. It might be very mild range of motion exercises for your joints. For the bariatric surgery, it might be that losing a little bit of weight before you go will help keep the surgery in the ambulatory care centre as a day case, rather than an overnight stay in the hospital.

There is a weight cut-off point for a lot of ambulatory care centre bariatric surgeries; the surgeons won't operate if the client is above 350 pounds. Weighing less than 350 pounds reduces the possible complications with the anaesthetic, and allows the surgeon better access for the procedure. They also don't need to buy specialized equipment, such as beds, operating tables, and patient lifts which reduce their costs and keep the risks down for day surgery centre staff when transporting and moving clients. So there might be that discussion with you if you are slightly over their limit, they might want you to try and reduce your weight before you can actually proceed with the surgery as a day case.

Weight reduction or stopping medications prior to surgery, stopping smoking, special diet, new medications

Find out from the facility what kind of preparation work you'll need to do. They should give you some kind of list or worksheet for this as well. Depending on what the surgery is, you will need some preparation as I mentioned before, it may be breathing exercises, range of motion for joints or weight loss. For some surgeries such as dental or orthopaedics, you may be asked to start taking antibiotics prior to the surgery and you will need you doctor's support with this as they will need to prescribe them for you. Depending on where you are going, the facility might want you to take medications with you. Again, you will need to liaise with your doctor so you can get your prescription to take the required medications with you.

What vaccinations are required for international travel? Is there a Visa required?

You have to keep in mind that you are travelling abroad and you may need a Visa. If you need a Visa you should check what the Visa allows you to do while you are in the country, you may need a different visa if you are having surgery rather than a vacation. Also, with international travel you may need a series of vaccinations such as malaria, yellow fever, hepatitis A, hepatitis B, these will be dependent on where you are going.

Government of Canada website (http://travel. gc.ca/) states:

When travelling, you may be at risk for a number of vaccine preventable illnesses. Over time, the protection provided through vaccination against many illnesses may decrease. Your risk of getting certain diseases may also increase.

You should consult a health care provider or visit a travel health clinic preferably six weeks before you travel. This provides an opportunity to:

- review your immunization history
- make sure you are up-to-date according to your provincial/territorial immunization program
- discuss any health concerns you may have related to your trip

---

- assess your needs based on where you plan to travel and what you plan to do

Additional vaccines may be recommended depending on your age, planned travel activities and local conditions. Remember that preventing disease through vaccination is a lifelong process.

Some countries require proof that you have received a yellow fever vaccination, documented on an International Certificate of Vaccination or Prophylaxis before allowing you to enter the country. Without such proof, you may be refused entry, quarantine or vaccinated.

Some of these are a series of vaccinations, which means they might not be something you could have this week and travel next week. You might need lead-in time to have the vaccine series, and that will have to be included in the preparations of what you need to do before you go (just for the travel aspects of it). Again, remember, it's not just you: this will apply to you caregiver as well.

Government of Canada website; Medical tourism (http://travel.gc.ca/)

It is your responsibility to research the standards of the foreign health care facility and the licensing of the health care provider in your destination country. Find out how the medical services and facilities are accredited and how they are regulated. Verify the licensing of the facility or health professional and study any complaints, comments, reports and evaluations. Even if you research the facility and staff thoroughly, there is no guarantee that what you experience will match the information that you found.

Be aware of the implications of receiving medical care in other countries and be prepared. For example:

Some countries' medical services may not test blood for blood-borne infections like HIV or hepatitis B. There can also be a risk of acquiring malaria from local blood banks in areas where malaria is present. Avoid injections or blood transfusions except in an emergency.

Be aware that there are multi-drug resistant bacteria in hospitals and other health care facilities around the world.

Vulnerable people may be coerced into donating their organs without their full consent. As a result, "transplant tourism" and selling organs are illegal in many countries.

Packing, getting prepared, bringing medical supplies, reports, and x-rays

Are you being asked to bring medications with you? Do these include antibiotics or post-surgery meds? Find out and make a list.

Getting prepared to go on a trip and packing is often enough work on its own. However, you are going for surgery, so there's added stress and more things to consider and remember. This is the thing: depending on what you are having done a foreign facility may want you to bring your medications, antibiotics, post-surgery medicines or, a particular kind of dressing. You have to have that list of where you can get these items and the liaison between your doctors so you can actually get the prescription to get these medications before you go.

Of course, if they are asking you to take these kinds of things, especially if they start asking you to take dressings, I would definitely have another check of what the facility is like and why they can't provide the dressings that they are asking you to bring.

That's kind of a red flag. However, it may be innocent; it might be that there's a particular item on the market that they know you can get here that's wonderful for whatever you are having, and it's difficult to get there. However, it's always good to ask the, "why do I have to bring this?" questions.

Pack whatever you are going to need to make you feel good about cleanliness

We all have different levels of comfort and cleanliness including hand-cleaning items, linen and clothing. Make sure you take these items with you if you know you have preferences that will make you feel more comfortable.

This is travelling to another country. You don't want to get sick with something related to travel on top of the surgery you are going for. It's not just for you; this is for whoever's going with you as well. Ask if you can drink the water in the facility or are they going to provide water? What is it going to be like at the facility? Is there some food or drink item that you know makes you feel better if you are not feeling well? Can you take it with you just in case, if it may make all the difference? I mentioned earlier about pacing yourself when you arrive and not planning a hectic tourist schedule prior to your surgery. You also need to be careful with food. Don't stop at some roadside food stand the day before you are having surgery in case both you and your caregiver end up with some kind of gastric upset and your surgery has to be cancelled.

Your post-surgery needs: will they be provided or should you bring it with you?

You want to be as comfortable as you can after your surgery. Make sure that in addition to any items the facility has asked you to bring with you, that you have the right kind of comfortable clothes during your recovery. Think ahead and ask questions about what you'll be able to do after your surgery. You have to really plan this; it's not a holiday, its surgery. It is somewhere that you are not familiar with, so the more that you can bring that can facilitate the comfort aspect of your post-surgery days, the better. And, of course, the mindset that this is all going to be great and you are really engaged in the whole process will really help, too.

You never realize how much is not available in other countries until you are there and you can't get what you are used to getting here. It could be as simple as you can't start your day without a particular coffee, tea or cereal. If you know that, take it with you. This is going to make the difference for you feeling good at the start of the day. If you know that whenever you have toast you need a particular kind of marmalade or jam take it with you. Anything you can do that's going to make it easier and more familiar for you.

What type of safeguards do you need to take?

It's a trip abroad; you need to make all the regular travel precautions and safety steps. For example make sure you have got the right type of Visa and that your money's going to be safe. In what form are you going to take your money? Are you going to take travelers' cheques? What about cash? How much do you need? What's going to happen when you are in the hospital? Will you be going back to the same hotel or is it a different room? Can you leave items in the hotel safe? Does the place where you have left your passport, your Visa, and your money feel safe?

If you have time before your surgery to explore a bit, depending on where you are, it might be that you shouldn't be wandering around on your own, and you will need someone with you. If you are going to go site seeing or shopping, talk to the hotel or the hospital ask if they provide a service that you can use. Don't just wander around somewhere and think that you can just flag down a cab down, especially if you don't speak the language.

Arrival plan B: What do you do if you just don't feel confident that this is for you after you arrive?

Do you have an option to opt-out or defer the surgery? What happens if after you arrive you are not confident in the plans you have made?

This is definitely a question you need to ask before you go, especially if you are someone that's not used to travelling, and if the country you have chosen is going to be completely out of your realm of experience. You may be in a completely different culture, with sights, sounds and smells that are very foreign to you. What do you do if you get there and you just do not feel comfortable and you can't go through with it? Is there someone you will be able to speak to and say, "I can't do this; it's just going to have to be a holiday"? What can you do rather than just sucking it up and going through with it? If you enter into the surgery with an uneasy mindset, you won't get the outcome you expect.

What are the ramifications of opting out?

Can it be turned into just a holiday? What happens in terms of payment?

If someone gets there and, for some reason, they are not going through with the surgery, is there the option for them to turn into a vacation if this is an elective surgery and they are well enough to continue without having the surgery? What happens about the money that has been paid for the surgery? Is there a minimum deduction? What happens if you can't go through with it or if, for some reason, it needs to be delayed? If you get there and you decide you can't go through with it or you are not well, if something happens that you can't have that surgery such as, the flight's upset you in some way These are all questions that need to be asked prior to you leaving the country and arriving at the facility.

Psychological see-saw effect is normal; how do you handle the stress?

You are not going to feel normal when you get there. There is a lot to consider when you are travelling. You'll probably be in a different time-zone, and be three, five, eight hours ahead or behind your usual timeframe. Also, who knows how long you have been travelling; you might have had at least one, if not two, stopovers on the flight, which may have been several hours added on to your travel. Your body has to adjust to all of that. Then there's the question, are you a good traveler to start with or, is your caregiver? Some people just don't travel well or they don't like planes. You might be someone who actually can't go on a plane and can only travel by car, bus or train. That will limit your choices for medical tourism destinations. For example, you might opt to go to Mexico because you can drive there. It adds to the psychological emotional side of making the decision for surgery abroad.

Is the travelling aspect of this going to stress you out? Add that to the dynamic of being in pain, going for surgery. How are you going to manage that stress?

Proximity to other passengers on buses and trains can be more of a problem as the spaces are more cramped that on planes and the journeys can be longer. There's documented evidence that 13 passengers and crew from a train in China were exposed to A (H1N1) virus by a passenger who made the 40 hour trip while sick with the virus.

22% to 64% of people who travel to developing countries report some health problem, and each day abroad increases the chances of illness 3-4%

Asia accounted for 55% of all new cases of TB in 2009; the World Health Organization classifies Brazil, India and Thailand as high burden countries for endemic TB.

Unseen Travellers: Medical Tourism and the spread of Infectious Disease

Hodges and Kimball 2012

A New Experience Outside Your Comfort Zone.

You may find that the drive from the airport to your wonderful five-star hotel or hospital, might take you past ghettos, where the children are playing in the dirt or running beside the taxi begging for money. This can be a real shock and eye-opener for some people. You are going there and you will be saving money, and suddenly, you see the dire poverty right next to where you are going. Literally, it can be right next door. I was reading an article that stated that the laborers who were building a hospital especially for medical tourism wouldn't actually be allowed go to the hospital they were building. Their relatives would have to continue the practice of loading them onto a cart and taking them half a day's walk to get them medical assistance if they are hurt or sick because, they are not allowed in the new hospital.

Hopefully, you will not be exposed to this ethical dilemma, I have heard of a story where the person going for a kidney transplant did not go through with it as it wasn't until she arrived in the country that she realised the impact her surgery was having on the local people. Three generations of families where known to have donated a kidney in an attempt to improve their lifestyle and younger family members were waiting eagerly to the time when they were old enough to donate.

On the day of your surgery, do you know what will actually happen?

Do you have a detailed itinerary for the whole process from arrival, pre-surgery, surgery, post-operation and recovery days? You should be aware of the entire plan for both you and your caregiver before you go. When you arrive, there will probably be someone from the facility to meet you at the airport and will either be taken to a hotel before you visit the facility, or you will go to the facility and do all the prep. Usually, you will be taken to a hotel to allow you some downtime and time to settle in. Depending on the surgery you are having, it is usually scheduled for one or two days after you arrive, so you'll probably be staying overnight at the prior to your surgery. On the morning of your surgery, a taxi or a mini-bus will pick you up and take you to the places you need to be. Perhaps you need tests or assessments, and there will be the face-to-face consultation with your surgeon. Quite often, there's someone who will escort you from the facility. Your caregiver should accompany you for any surgery related meetings; they need to know exactly what you have been told so they can be a good advocate if you are unable to communicate after surgery.

If you will be staying overnight in the facility after your surgery will your caregiver be staying with you in the hospital, or will they go back to the hotel? Is the caregiver's transportation to the hotel and back the next day arranged? You don't want to be worrying about what's happening with your caregiver when you come out of surgery.

Are there conversations with the doctors beforehand?

You will probably have spoken to your surgeon by phone or on Skype, prior to leaving for the facility. Usually you would see the surgeon or another doctor when you arrive so they can examine you in person. You should also see someone about the anaesthetic you are having and there should be an examination to ensure that you are okay for the proposed anaesthetic. Depending on the type of surgery, it might be a nurse who discusses the anesthetic procedure with you. Regardless, there should definitely be some face-to-face meetings with healthcare providers who are going to be dealing with you for the surgery.

Where does the caregiver fit into it all?

This is very important, because your caregiver is going to be your intermediary. You will probably be shown your room and have an introduction to the surgery process. Your caregiver needs to know what else is available at that site; obviously they are going to have time to fill while you are in having the surgery, so they'll want to know what's available at the location or if they will return to the hotel and wait. They will also need to get their bearings: where is the nurses' station? What if they want to talk to someone? Do they speak the language and is there a contact number they can call? Quite often, clients having surgery abroad are given cell phones upon arriving. The phones have pre-programed numbers so you can instantly dial for help if you have a query or a problem. You speed-dial the number, and it will get you through to someone that speaks your language and they can sort out any problems that have arisen. Cell phones like these are essential when you arrive, especially if the facility staff doesn't speak the language.

If you are having the bariatric surgery, you'll probably be in the ambulatory surgery unit for the day and then you'll go back to the hotel (day surgery). If you are having orthopedic surgery, you'll stay in the hospital for a few days at least. Then it's a question of, is your caregiver going to stay with you? Quite often, these rooms are big enough that the caregiver will stay in the room with you. Usually, there's a trundle bed but in the more deluxe facilities, the room is similar to a hotel suite with a full size bed for your caregiver.

The recovery stage

Depending on the type of surgery you have, it may be necessary to have a drain(s) inserted to allow any body fluids accumulated after the surgery to drain away. This is particularly the case with orthopedic surgery where you'll probably have at least one drain. In the pre-surgery conversation with the facility staff or the surgeon, you will have been made aware that you are going to wake up with drains hanging out of your incision site. There should be a plan for the drain and the dressing to be checked while you are in the facility. If you still have the drain and dressing in place when you are discharged to a hotel, you have to find out that the nurse is going to come at least every day and check on the drainage.

You also need to be aware of when your physiotherapy will start. Some hip surgeries require you to get up on the day of your surgery. You should ask if you should be up and about. These details should all be sorted out beforehand and worked out with your caregiver: how much can they actually do to assist you when the nurse or the physiotherapist is not there? Your caregiver should have some definite input into this, to make sure they are able to provide the assistance needed and to be encouraging and helping you. After all, that's what they are there for. If your caregiver is going to be assisting you with standing, or transferring from the bed to a chair, make sure they are shown how to do it properly. The last thing you need is your caregiver straining their back or pulling you the wrong way and affecting your recovery.

Is a nurse coming in to check dressings, or do you go to the hospital? What happens to your sutures?

Usually, the nurses, I'm told, come every day, to check your dressings, and your sutures will be removed while you are at the hotel. You will probably be assigned one nurse which provides familiarity and consistency, for you and in the observation of your drain and dressing. The doctor may also come to the hotel to see you. Definitely your dressings and drains will be checked. Sutures may need to be removed, they might be dissolvable or they might be staples, and that will all probably be dealt with at the hotel by a nurse from the facility.

Have you arranged for physio while you are there? When is it? Where?

Whether exercises are necessary will depend on the type of surgery you have had. You will want to be up and moving as soon as possible to prevent any respiratory complications or DVT occurring. You should be doing the breathing exercises you were taught before your surgery to expand your lungs fully. If you have had joint surgery, the physiotherapist will often visit you at your hotel. Sometimes you'll be a few days at the hotel and then if you have booked convalescence in the package, you might move to another hotel affiliated with the facility, which specializes in convalescence and recuperation. The physiotherapy will probably continue at that hotel as well.

When are you leaving? Who decides that you are fit to travel?

You need to make sure the sutures and drains are out, the incision site is healing well, and that you can walk properly before your journey home. You must see the surgeon and get the final sign-off before you are discharged from the facility. You should also have an estimate of the time when you can return home. To make this experience as seamless as possible there should be a plan B. What will you do if your recovery isn't as fast as anticipated or there is something that sets back your recovery? What leeway do you have regarding taking extra time and money needed to recover fully? If you have drains or a suture line that you are having a problem with, what's the alternative plan to ensure you have a safety net and are fit to travel?

Element Five: Coming Home and Sharing the Best Possible Outcome

What do they need to bring back with you?

WHEN YOU ARE coming home, you need to have an operation report; which would include details of the actual surgery you had. It should also include the drugs you have been given, through the course of treatment, and any antibiotics you might be on. The reports should include the type of anaesthetic you had, whether it was local, regional or general, so your healthcare practitioners, when you get back, have the full picture of everything you were given as far as medication, and the procedures you had when you were away.

It should be written in your primary language; French, English, whatever you speak, so that when you come back and give these reports to your health professional, they can read them straight away. You don't want something in Spanish when you and your healthcare practioner speak French or English. It needs to be a report in the language that you speak and it needs to be exactly what the procedure was that you had done.

This is very important for continuity and follow-up

Continuity of treatment and follow-up is very important in the event that you do have anything out of the ordinary happen to you when you arrive home, like a rash or a skin reaction, and you think it's not is related to the surgery site. It may be that when looking through the documentation, your doctor realizes you are having a reaction to one of the medications given while you were away. Unless the doctor has the complete list of medications and anaesthetics you have been given, when you present to them with symptoms, rash, inflammation, swelling they won't know what you are having a reaction to. They need a baseline. You might have an allergy to latex, which could be in the gloves or the tape used when changing your dressing; it could be kind of dressing, the salve or powder used as part of the dressing. If there's no documentation of what's been given or applied to you, it's very difficult to start appropriate treatment in a timely manner and, depending in the problem you are having, there could be serious effects caused by the delay in identifying the source of the problem.

Aftercare; what's happening when you get home.

Once you return home, and depending on the kind of surgery you have had, you may be on medications, maybe antibiotics. You will need to keep an eye on the surgical incision site, to make sure that nothing is happening to delay the healing process and to ensure that you don't get an infection. Your incision could be very minimal, just a couple of little incisions if you have had for minimally-invasive surgery, which might be covered with a Band-Aid. Or it might be you had an Orthopaedic surgery and you have returned home with a very extensive dressing on the site.

If you return home with a dressing in place, how are you going to look after it, or who is looking after it for you? Is someone coming to check on it? These are things that need to be arranged prior to going for surgery, and should all be scheduled to begin as soon as you return. When you are home, you are still going to have a fresh scar, and will want to be keeping track of how it's healing.

With medical tourism and travel, sometimes timeframes might be cut a little short due to costs. It's very important when you are coming home to ensure that there is continuity of care.

Checking into the standards of aftercare and expected recovery time here.

Before you go abroad for your surgery you should make sure that you check what the usual aftercare and recovery time is, as if you had the surgery here. You can do that by either asking your health practitioner, or by checking with the hospital and their website for information and checklists. Your doctor, will hopefully, be on board with you getting this surgery, and should be able to give you information of what to expect. The hospital-provided information sheets and checklists describe pre-surgery and post-surgery procedures. They will give you an expectation of what's usually happening after your type of surgery and what kind of follow-up there would be.

When you are having a procedure abroad, you are taking matters into your own hands. To a certain degree, you can't make any assumptions you'll be cared for in the way you would be if the procedure were done at home. That being the case there is a need for you to have a more in-depth understanding of the procedure and what is required afterwards to aid your speedy recovery.

The audience for medical tourism is much more engaged and the participants far more proactive. With that in mind, you can't leave anything up to chance or make any assumptions. Ask lots of questions and don't assume that it's going to be like surgery done at home.

Follow up with the surgeon from the facility to see how you are.

It's very important that the surgeon actually gives you the okay to travel, because traveling home too early could be detrimental to your recovery. At the discharge consultation you need to ensure that you get all the information regarding what medications and follow up will be necessary and for how long. If you are on a course of antibiotics, it's very important that you finish the entire course of antibiotics. Don't just stop taking them when you leave the country because the prophylactic (prevention of infection) intention of the antibiotics won't work unless the complete course is taken.

During the discharge consultation you need to confirm with the surgeon that you are going to be safe when flying home. Remember, that if you are having gastric surgery, the air pressure in the plane can affect the gasses in your gut and, depending on the surgery you have had that can be a problem. It's very important to get the okay from the surgeon to fly home, especially if it's going to be a very long flight.

Surgeries and healing. Planning and schedules.

The healing and the need for basic aftercare may require a very flexible schedule based on the patient's response to drugs and procedures. The more compliant you are and the more positive your attitude the faster your recovery will be. You won't have the kind of recovery that is expected if you have been told that you have to follow a particular diet and, do particular exercises, but do not follow that regime. Basically, you need to be compliant with your recovery plan, including your drugs, and exercise regime otherwise, the expected healing timeline won't fit into the recovery schedule.

Ensuring medical follow-up and continuity at home

Prior to booking your surgery abroad make sure your medical practitioner at home is agreeable, so you know that when you come back, you can go and see them with all the related documents, and you can say, "Okay, this is what I had done; these are the drugs I'm on and, this is the plan they've given me for physiotherapy or diet afterward."

You don't want any surprises when you return home. You need to know you've got a doctor who's willing to look after you, especially if you have had extensive or life changing surgery. You want to ensure that you have a medical practitioner that's going to see you through the recovery stage.

If something goes wrong, can you go back to the facility or get it dealt with here?

We never know how somebody will respond to surgery or how a procedure will go, because we can't predict 100%. There are basic, common sense observations regarding a surgical incision. You should be keeping tabs on whether you are feeling more pain than you anticipated, whether there's any swelling or excessive bruising. Also, after surgery note whether you are getting headaches that you don't usually have, be aware of any unusual symptoms so you can mention them to your surgeon, hopefully before you leave the country. There are no stupid questions; ask them all! "Is this right? I noticed that there is more bruising today," or "I'm getting these headaches; is that okay?" This is important because all of these things could be related to a minor complication with the surgical site, or it could be something to do with the anesthetic you were given. As with any surgery, these are the signs and symptoms you should be aware of: inflammation, nausea and vomiting. Therefore make sure that you are mentioning these to your healthcare practitioner don't try to tough things out.

When you set up the contract for your surgery remember to ask about total costs. What if there was a complication after the surgery? Would the facility deal with that as part of that procedure, or are you going to be charged again? How many days after surgery does the facility cover?

Any time you have a procedure done, it's good to have continual follow-up from the surgeon who knows your condition and knows how things went with the procedure. However, having your surgery abroad means you will not have that continuity of care because you come home. An example of being proactive with this might be regarding your incision site. Most cell phones have cameras, which would allow you to take photos of your incision site to record how it's healing. You can then use the photos as a reference, when you are back. If it looks a bit different when someone's doing the dressing, you can show them the photo and say, "Well, this is what it looked like the last day that I was abroad." The photos will give a baseline; a frame of reference for whoever is continuing with your treatment here to work with.

Instant gratification may play a large role in your decision to have your surgery abroad.

With the websites and all the marketing, you can basically click on the surgeries and add-ons you want; it's almost like being in the candy store: it's instantaneous! We live in a culture where instant gratification is a high expectation. If you have the money you can get whatever you want, whenever you want. That's why, given our healthcare system here along with its timeframes, instant gratification might be a big factor for why you are going abroad for surgery.

The instant gratification factor also plays into the medical tourism "upsell", *that extra procedure that you may as well have while you're here;* especially when it comes to cosmetic or dental treatments. You might go for two root canals and then end up agreeing to have several unplanned procedures such as veneers, crowns, or possibly even implants. It's not what you anticipated, but it will be within a good price range. You will probably still be saving money however, do you really need all the work done, especially in a short time frame? Think of all the time that you will spend in the dentist chair. With so many procedures carried out at one time, how will you know if your swelling or puffiness afterwards is normal? When should you be going to see someone if you have a problem? Have you already started travelling home or arrived home? Will your regular dentist see you? Do you wait too long before going to your dentist because you are embarrassed to admit the extent of the work you had done abroad? How will that affect the recovery time?

What do you need now and what appointments do you need scheduled

You have to remember the timelines and constraints of our healthcare system in this country, versus your needs that are suddenly imposed upon it because you came back from surgery abroad and need the aftercare. If you haven't made arrangements, you may encounter big gaps in treatment while you wait for your appointments. It's not just arranging everything to go abroad to have this surgery, you also really have to pay as much attention to the follow up arrangements when you are back. It may be that you have been wanting this surgery for quite a while and suddenly you find out you can have it abroad in two weeks' time. In your eagerness to get it done as soon as possible, you must remember there are a lot of arrangements that need to be made for your return. Getting these to fit in with timetables on this end will probably play a role in when and where you schedule your surgery, or in what timeframe it can all happen.

Also, you have got to consider how you are going to get to these appointments. Who's going to help you out? Anyone having surgery feels pretty rough afterwards for a few days however, on top of that, you'll have had surgery abroad, you'll have stayed for a recovery period for however many days (or if you are lucky, however many weeks you are able to stay there) then you will have to fly back. Any jet lag will compound all the other post-surgical feelings that you'll have, so you have to remember to build it and returning from abroad into your recovery plans.

Rehab and Recover Specific to Desired Outcomes

A lot of the arrangements you normally assume will be handled for you are now becoming your responsibility. You have to know what kinds of arrangements need to be made because you don't have that hospital machine following its process for you.

Post-surgery, you might not be as mobile, so it's not only arranging these appointments, it's determining how you are going to get to them. If you can't get to the pharmacy to pick up your prescription, who will go and get it for you or will the pharmacy deliver? Day to day practicalities need to be thought through and built into your plans.

Leaving your surgeon in another country means you don't have the person with the judgment or experience to offer guidance in the same way as when your surgeon's here, or when your practitioners are all here. That's why many medical tourism facilities utilize Skype for patients to access the surgeon after they return home. Also phone numbers are often provided where you can speak directly to the surgeon. You should ask about these types of follow up services when researching your surgery facility.

It may be possible for the surgeon abroad to connect with your doctor for continuity when you come back. They'll be talking the same language when it comes to terminology, procedures and medicines. It may also be possible for your healthcare practitioner to contact your surgeon if they have concerns or questions about your case. Check with the facility about surgeon to doctor conference calls.

What are the considerations in timeframe for a complete recovery?

What limitations are there in terms of working or time off or modification of duties? This is something that you should be discussing before you go, either with your healthcare practitioner at home or the surgeon abroad. You have got to have a timeline, because depending on the surgery that you have, you will need to get the timeframe of when you can be thinking of going back to work. For example, if you go for plastic surgery on your nose, it's going to be a different timeframe than if you have surgery for a knee replacement. You'll also need to know whether you need a gradual return to work and its length, or whether you'll actually be able to return to work and do your full duties. It may be that during the time t you were waiting for your knee replacement, you were doing a job with physical modifications. So will you be going back to your original job? You have to sort out all of those details with your workplace.

Physiotherapy: what do you need, how much, where, and who?

You will want to be going to a physiotherapist who specializes in recovery after the type of procedure you have had. . Having knowledge of who the experts are in your speciality beforehand and getting on their waiting list or getting scheduled with them would be an important factor in scheduling your procedure. Also, you might have to travel. There might not be someone in your area that does exactly what you need to enhance your recovery. This is research you need to do before your surgery.

Diet and nutrition: Helps the body to heal

If you are going to be having surgery, you need to be at your peak of health because, whether it's a small surgery or a major one, this will aid your healing and recovery. You should really be reviewing your diet before any surgery to make sure you can be as strong and energized as possible. It might be that if you are having gastric surgery there's a particular diet that you should be on or you might need to lose a bit of weight before you have the surgery. Losing weight might be a requirement, as some bariatric surgeries, are carried out in an ambulatory care, as a day surgery. Often these facilities often won't operate on people if they are more than 350 pounds, because that's their safety limit for a day surgery patient. Therefore, it might be that you have to lose those extra pounds before the procedure can be done. With any elective surgery if you are a bit overweight, try and lose some weight and try to increase your exercise as much as possible. This will help optimize your respiratory and circulatory systems. If you smoke, quit prior to your surgery and do exercises to practice how to breathe deeply to allow your lungs to expand properly after the surgery. The more information you have, and the more prepared you can be physically and mentally, the better outcome you are going to have.

Psychosocial support necessary for your recovery

When it comes to surgery, you are going to feel like you are pushing a rock up a hill if you haven't got the support of your family, friends and peers. If you say to someone, "I'm going abroad and I'm going to have this surgery", and their response is very negative it will be very demoralizing for you, especially if they are your main support. You will need all the psychological and physical support you can get when you return home. Depending on the type of surgery, you will need to have buy-in with your decision, that yes, you are having this surgery, yes, you are going to need physical help, yes, you are going to need that emotional support when you come back because this is surgery; this is potentially a life changing event.

Making the Perfect Outcome a Reality

Visualize the outcome you wanted this surgery to create, and see it perfectly. This is the mindset piece of the puzzle; why things work so well for some people and not so well for others.

You have to be focused on what you want, but you have to also be realistic. You might have had a problem with your joints for many years and are excited for the surgery to fix the problem, but you still, have to have the reality check that this surgery isn't magically going to allow you to run marathons. However, at the same time, you have to have a vision of the outcome you want to achieve so you can work towards that vision. If you are having plastic surgery, you have to have realization that this is what you have visualized you will look like afterwards. This is the physical form that you desire, and what it will be like afterwards. It's setting realistic goals and expectations, before the surgery.

Sometimes people think the surgery is magic and it's going to make everything perfect immediately. However, you have to consider the timeframe in which you'll see the improvement.

Setting small goals; making it realistic so you stay positive.

You have to do the work after the surgery by taking the medications, doing the physiotherapy, following the exercise regime, and changing your eating habits, if necessary. You also have to be realistic in that you may have some bruising and won't be able to see results straight away. You'll have to pace yourself and not look for the instant gratification that we're all getting so used to these days and know that it does take some time to see results.

Depending on the surgery, it might be a matter of days, or it might be weeks before you see improvement. Be realistic. Each day you should notice some positive change; "Oh, I can do more of this," or "The swelling's gone down, the bruising's gone down, I'm feeling better." "This looks better." Take notice of those small steps forward so you can still remain positive. It may also help to keep a journal of the whole process.

Noticing the impact of the surgery on your life and how it has changed.

That's what you are really looking for: a better life.

Write down your goals and expectation. List the things you plan to do; you are going to be able to reach that goal by this date. Plan small or short-term treats for when you've reached each goal, such as getting a particular outfit you have wanted, or returning to a sport you enjoy, or taking part in a sport you haven't been able to participate in before. Having realistic goals, set out in small achievable sections will aid your recovery.

You have a big role in the outcome you desire, and you must be persistent to achieve it; the surgery is only a little piece of it. It's not magic, there's no magician waving his wand at you; it's actually a scalpel! You play a huge part in this process. It's all to do with the mindset you have, how physically engaged you are in the process, and the optimum health you can achieve prior to the surgery. It's also following through with the physical and emotional effort that's needed during recovery. The ultimate goal is that you believe this procedure is going to make you happier or give you a better quality of life.

Living the Life and Enjoying the Outcome

What can you do that you could not do before?

This can depend on the level of surgery you are having. It could be that you have had some plastic surgery and now you feel confident that you can go into social situations that you couldn't go into before, or you feel it might help your career. If it's an Orthopaedic surgery, you can now be up and moving, whereas before, perhaps you had a more sedentary lifestyle. The surgery offers you possibilities that you couldn't have without it. It gives you an ability to move forward and achieve some of the goals you've planned.

Building the life you want starts with achieving your small goals. Within a month of returning home, plan to do something you would not have been able to do before you had this surgery. Again, don't make it too big; you don't want to over-extend yourself. It should be something you have got to aim for, by a certain date. Maybe plan something three months down the road to take the kids and do something you haven't been able to do before. It's very important to have set goals to achieve.

Celebrating the achievements along the way

It really does make things go better when we focus on and are appreciative of any improvements. I think the big change for a lot of people after they've gone for surgery is being pain-free. A lot of the contributing factors will have been focused on pain, and once you don't have that pain anymore, the change in people is phenomenal. To be released from pain and be more mobile; that's definitely something to celebrate!

Healing beyond your expectations and allowing this to be life-changing

Getting ahead of the curve by doing your research and going abroad to have, this surgery done, then going through the healing process is really part of the celebration. Now you should be going out there and doing more in life than you have done before. You have gone through all of this process, so make the most of it. Don't fall back into bad habits with eating or not exercising. Get out there and do it!

There's so much to be learned when you do take matters into your own hands and you are proactive about what you want. Remember the woman who became the advocate for gastric surgery and how making the decision to have surgery herself led her to completely change her life and move forward to help others. People can create even bigger outcomes than they imagined.

For some people it will be the mere fact they have traveled abroad to have this surgery. Traveling abroad can be life-changing. It may be the first time you have left the country and could possibly encourage you to travel again. Some health insurance companies are now giving people the option of traveling abroad to have surgeries done instead of at home, and there are a lot of people in this group who have never, ever been abroad. When you were looking at this surgery and if you arranged it yourself, you likely learned all kinds of information you had never considered before. You might be a traveler, however, you might not have been to the particular country where your surgery was performed. You may also have seen parts of the country that tourists don't often see and were able to interact with staff that live in the culture. It will expand your life experience, as traveling always expands our life anyway. You meet different people, are exposed to different environments and it opens up your life.

Ask lots of questions and be safe!

Conclusion

THROUGHOUT THIS BOOK I have encouraged you to think about your choice of surgery abroad. I have asked you to ask questions of yourself, your family, and your healthcare providers here and abroad.

My hope is that this book will prompt you to consider previously unknown possibilities regarding the surgery that you are planning, and the location you are considering to travel for your surgery.

My intention is simple: to stimulate reflection and conversations about why you want the surgery abroad and what the effect on you, the healthcare system abroad, and at home may be in relation to your engagement in this venture.

My foremost hope is that you are safe, and achieve your desired outcome.

If you choose to go ahead with surgery abroad I'd like to hear from you about your experience, send an email to: janet@areusafe.ca

More information about medical tourism
can be found on my website:
areusafe.ca

26 Pre surgery Checklist questions

1. Why you are considering surgery abroad?
2. Do you know anyone who has had surgery abroad?
3. Does your regular doctor know you are planning this?
4. Do you have any pre-existing medical conditions which may impact a surgical procedure?
5. Will you be using a medical tourism facilitator to arrange this for you?
   a. Have they been recommended to you?
   b. How did you find them?
6. Do you know where you'd like to go for the surgery?
7. Why have you chosen this location?
   a. Have you been there before?
   b. Do you have family there?
   c. How long will it take to get to this destination?
8. Will you have someone accompanying you?
   a. Will they look after you post operation?
9. Do you know how much the surgery will cost?
   a. It is important to know what is included in any treatment costs quoted, make sure that you understand exactly what is included.
10. Do you know which facility / surgeon you would prefer?

11. What do you know about the facility you're going to?

12. Does the facility specialize in medical tourism?

    a. How long have they seen patients from abroad?

13. Does the facility specialize in the surgery you're looking for?

    a. What medical records will be needed for the pre-surgery consultation; X-rays, blood tests recent doctors notes

14. Who will be your surgeon?

    a. Will they personally be performing the surgery and overseeing your care?

15. Where did the surgeon train? What are their credentials?

    a. a surgeon should be actively engaged in their speciality via association memberships and interested in keeping up international standards

16. How many of these surgeries have they performed recently?

    a. What is their infection rate?

    b. What happens if you have a problem post op?

17. Will you speak to the surgeon prior to travelling for the surgery?

18. Will you have access to the surgeon pre and post operation? (Phone number?)

    a. Will you have contact with the surgeon on your return to Canada?

    b. How long for?

19. How long will you stay in the country post operation?

20. Will you stay in the facility post operation or in a hotel?

    a. How near to the facility is the hotel?

21. Is the facility accredited?

    a. What was their accreditation status?

22. Do they have their own a Medical Device Reprocessing Department (MDRD) on site?

    a. How are their MDRD staff trained?

23. Where are the Operating Room staff, anaesthetists and nurses trained?

24. Will you be provided a legible copy of your operation notes (in English/French) for your doctor and follow up care back home?

25. What if you get an infection or complication when you arrive home?

26. Will your regular doctor continue to treat you when you return?

    a. If not who will be looking after you?

CPSIA information can be obtained
at www.ICGtesting.com
Printed in the USA
LVOW04s2155290116

472894LV00025B/752/P